CONTENTS

KU-678-956

$\mathcal{P}$REFACE

AUTHOR'S NOTE

My initial doubts and queries regarding reflexology have over
the years led to many questions and much in-depth research
which, with the wisdom of previous masters and philosophers,
my colleagues, therapists, students and friends, has unearthed
the true nature and value of reflexology.

This book contains universal knowledge that, to many, is pure
common sense! Its contents have been channelled through for
the benefit of mankind and it is offered with unconditional love,
sincerity and joy.

Our wellbeing relies on the balanced state of a healthy mind,
body and soul. Physiologically, the body outwardly expresses
personal sentiments and perceptions of the mind, arising from
profound, individual feelings of the soul.

Thoughts of love, joy and acceptance, on every level,
produce overall harmony, whereas distress creates emotional
havoc. Long-term, inner turmoil from unresolved issues, that are
consciously suppressed into the subconscious mind, erupt in the
form of dis-ease, unless dealt with on a conscious or
subconscious level.

In this book, the reader is encouraged to look beyond
physical irritants as being the cause of illness, and recognise
festering emotions to be the basis of dis-comfort and dis-ease
within the self. Strong reactions are likely, especially amongst
those who are understandably afraid to acknowledge their true
feelings, since the truth can stir old hurts. This is where
reflexology steps in! By composing the mind, relaxing the body
and boosting the whole, the reader can competently face life's
challenges with an inner calm.

May it bring peace, health, happiness and prosperity to all.

*i*NTRODUCTION

Reflexology's increasing popularity worldwide is due to its extraordinary effectiveness in maintaining good health as well as relieving all forms of physical and mental discomfort. Its far-reaching effects stem from the deep state of relaxation that creates space for the mind, body and soul to heal themselves.

The body has no power or inclination to generate dis-ease. Stress does not enter the body, but is manufactured from within, making it vulnerable and susceptible to physical and emotional disorders.

In its natural state, the body enjoys full health. Instinctive survival means that subjectively the subconscious and unconscious minds are capable of a multitude of life-saving functions but, objectively, the mind obeys conscious choices that generally plunge it into a world of doubt, confusion, frustration and anger. Blood vessels contract and the body, deprived of essential life forces, feels 'ill at ease'.

Reflexology reverses the process by expelling suppressed emotions that hamper progress and weigh down the body. The body is released from the shackles of self-constraint and social restriction and new vibrant energies are directed along natural pathways to untangle energy congestion and stagnation. Rejuvenation and revitalisation can be immediately experienced.

Bodily tissue has an amazing capacity to regenerate itself. In natural circumstances, cells remain innately healthy. Through reflexology a conducive environment for the regeneration of healthy vibrant cells is created.

Reflexology has until recently been practised on a purely physical basis. However, with the rapid shift in consciousness, in which the physical state is widely acknowledged to reflect the emotional mind, a more 'wholistic' approach incorporating mind, body and soul has proved invaluable.

In our current rushed, highly demanding life, reflexology has had to keep pace and provide an antidote to the continual build-up of tension, anxiety and fear.

This *Definitive Guide* offers detailed suggestions for the immediate relief from most forms of discomfort through the stimulation of the appropriate reflexes in the feet. It also mentions other forms of healing that can enhance and accelerate the healing process.

As nature's gift to mankind, reflexology is instinctively simple and has no detrimental side effects, especially if sensitively and empathetically administered.

Furthermore, the book offers a deeper insight into the nature and cause of dis-orders and dis-ease. Used between professional reflexology treatments and alongside other forms of treatment, health and well-being will be enhanced.

The only limiting factor is ourselves. We need to overcome the current epidemic of self doubt that has arisen from the unjust appraisal and evaluation of human worth and stop being so judgemental and critical of ourselves and others. It is not the world that needs healing, but our thoughts and belief systems, because mankind is destroying itself through a lack of love and faith.

It is time to stop blaming the physical world and others for our misfortunes and to look within. We can choose to sit out in the cold and complain bitterly, or we can choose a life that contains all the elements of happiness.

There are no chemical cures for emotional injuries and surgery cannot remove painful hurts!

Reflexology enriches the quality of life, by providing the confidence to express the self with love and honesty, the strength to face life's challenges without emotional upset and by releasing us from the frustration of having to pretend to be the person others expect us to be!

A similarity can be drawn to an electric light bulb. By touching a switch in one part of the room, a bulb is activated elsewhere, but the whole environment is affected and filled with light!

Use this book to step ahead with joy and confidence and achieve your highest potential! There is no better time to begin than now!

*t*HE LAYOUT OF THE GUIDE

Definition

A physical explanation and description of a specific bodily system, part or dis-ease.

Emotional aspect

Related emotions that may cause the imbalance and trigger off physical dis-ease. Since several similar emotions can make the body feel uneasy, more than one suggestion may be mentioned, although only one may apply.

Reflexes

- The main reflexes to be stimulated for each particular condition.
- No matter whether servicing an already healthy body, or easing a specific dis-ease or ailment, all reflexes on both feet should always be thoroughly massaged to stimulate the whole.
- Specific reflexes, that if given *extra* attention, will enhance the healing process.
- For specified ailments, always refer to the reflexes mentioned uder the general systemic dis-orders at the beginning of each section.
- Many reflexes overlap, eg: nerve, circulatory and lymphatic reflexes, and are repeatedly mentioned to indicate their importance in keeping the body toxin-free.
- This is truly a guide, since individuals respond differently to a particular dis-ease. If during massage it is felt that an unmentioned reflex requires extra attention, then intuitively follow your instincts.
- Individuals constantly change and so too should the massage. There are times when a firmer approach is preferred to the lighter touch. The best way to administer reflexology is to 'tune' in and instinctively respond to individual requirements.

3

- Direct reflexes are generally mentioned. If these are too sensitive to the touch, approach from the secondary reflex, on the immediate opposite side of the foot, for example breast reflexes can be directly stimulated on the balls of the feet or indirectly from the corresponding position on top of the feet.
- Rigidity in the feet indicates rigidity in the body, whilst flexible feet support a flexible body. By easing tension in the feet through massage and manipulation, tension can be expelled from the body. Stroke, massage and gently manipulate the whole foot as often as possible throughout the treatment.
- Tension in the neck and shoulders restricts the flow of blood to and from the brain, hence the importance of always massaging these reflexes.
- Destructive emotions stored by the liver hamper progress. The release of these feelings through the massage of the liver reflexes creates space for new vibrant, healthy cells.
- Whenever treating a child, treat the parents as well. Children reflect parental subconscious moods and feelings long before the parents themselves are aware of their own emotions!
- When a person is severely ill, treat also the loved ones to give them the strength and understanding to deal with the extra demands.

Other suggestions

Practical tips that provide a variety of options. Those that are particularly relevant to a certain disease are mentioned in the text, but also refer to Other Suggestions under general ailments of each bodily system. However, any of the following can be used for most conditions.

Seek professional guidance
- This includes a host of specialists: homoeopath, naturopath, general practitioner, herbalist, acupuncturist, osteopath, chiropractor, physiotherapist, reflexology therapist, aromatherapist, podiatrist, speech therapist, music therapist, dietician, and so on.
- Individuals will know who, for them, is the professional best

able to guide them in their particular circumstances.
- True professionals guide rather than advise providing the individual with a basis and choice of what, for them, is the best way to heal themselves.

Details of support groups
- Generally these organisations are formed by people who, with first-hand knowledge and experience of specific ailments, are able to provide appropriate support and useful suggestions.
- Where no address is given, contact your local authority.

Local authorities, health visitors and social workers
- Will provide: Information and arrangements for necessary support such as disability benefits, aids, meals-on-wheels, home help, rehabilitation groups, transport, financial assistance and so on.
- The health visitor will also visit the home to see whether adjustments can be made to improve the quality of life.

Aromatherapy essential oils
- Enhances the effects of reflexology, especially when they are massaged into the feet. Essential oils and their aromas are immediately absorbed from the feet and distributed throughout the whole.
- For a foot or body massage, use one to three drops of one or more of the oils mentioned, diluted with 30 ml of vegetable oil.
- Allow the recipient to decide which essential oils they would like, either by choosing the bottle(s) with the left hand, because this is the receptive and receiving side of the body, or through smell.
- Should there be a preference for an essential oil, other than those mentioned, use this as well, since there is obviously an innate need for its particular properties.
- Certain essential oils, extracted from herbs or fruits, for example ginger, thyme, basil, orange, lemon, can also be consumed in their edible form.
- Aromatherapy essential oils can also be used as follows:

for inhalation: mix one to two drops of one or more essential oils in a bowl with boiling water. Place on a stable surface. Cover the head and bowl with a small towel and take in large, deep breaths. Also place a drop of essential oil on a handkerchief or pillow.

in the bath: add one or two drops of the required aromatherapy oils mixed with 5 ml of vegetable oil, to the bath water.

in a burner: to infiltrate atmospheric air.

on a candle: for a relaxed, healing environment.

as a poultice: dip a cloth into warm water infused with the necessary essential oils, ring it out and then apply directly to the affected site.

as a mouthwash: dilute one drop of each suggested essential oil in a teaspoon of brandy and gargle. Do not swallow!

- If used sensitively and sensibly, aromatherapy oils can be safely used to enhance the effects of the reflexology massage.

Relaxation techniques to open the mind, relax the body and to get in touch with the true self

- *Hatha Yoga* for complete relaxation through specific bodily poses that naturally strengthen mind, body and soul. Join a local group with a qualified instructor.
- *Tai Chi*, increasingly popular in the Western world, to move energies through bodily movement to re-energise and fortify the whole.
- *Meditation* to relax the mind and establish contact with the higher self through the alpha state of consciousness. By stilling the mind and experiencing inner peace, there is greater understanding of the true self.
- *Deep breathing*. Lie on a flat surface, in a comfortable position, and slowly take in a deep breath, with a smile, savouring every molecule of air! Hold it for as long as is comfortable and then gradually release the breath until every last drop of air has been expelled. Hold it! Repeat as often as possible throughout the day. This is particularly beneficial in the bath!
- *Relaxation*. Listen to classical or soothing music.

Wholesome natural foods
- Food provides energy for activity and vibrancy for new cell formation. This energy is only available in natural raw foods.
- We are what we eat, *and* how we eat it!
- Aggression and anger immediately destroy any potential nutrients, so food should always be consumed in a tranquil environment with peace of mind.
- Balance is the key and if the body really needs a particular food, eat it!
- Food in itself is purely an energy.
- It is not the food that increases bodily weight, but the heavy emotions with which it is eaten.

Vitamin and mineral supplements
- To boost nutritional content or to fortify the body during times of vulnerability.
- Seek expert advice.

Drink plenty of purified water and natural, fresh fruit juices.
- Individual requirements vary considerably.
- The bulk of the body is water, so regular top-ups are necessary!
- Just like a stream, continuous movement prevents stagnation, keeping the water fresh, clean and clear of debris.

Visualisation
- Visualise specific parts, or the whole body, in a healthy vibrant state by taking thoughts within.
- Just as the face lights up with a smile, so it is that cell characteristics change with thoughts that spark hope and encouragement.

Oxygen or ozone therapy
- Based on the principle that since the body is mainly water, approximately 89 per cent of the body is oxygen! Depletion of this essential life force immediately distresses the body, creates havoc and cells malform.
- Regular deep breathing reverses this unnatural state of the body.
- Ozone therapy helps to destroy malformed cells especially in the case of AIDS and cancer since unnatural cells have difficulty in surviving in high levels of oxygen!

- For further information contact: Quantum Process, PO Box 184, East Kew, Victoria 3102, Australia (03) 810 9591.

Rebirthing
- Breath is held in perceivably life-threatening situations, whether real or imagined.
- From early childhood, many fears and anxieties are suppressed in this manner. Hence the expression 'Getting it off your chest'.
- These stumbling blocks to self-development and self-actualisation can be released through this natural breathing technique, allowing full expansion and expression of personal worth.

Massaging the auric space
- Even though physical bodily parts, such as a toe, may be missing, energies are still present.
- By massaging the image of the absent part, amazing results can be achieved.
- This can also apply to the space just beyond the physical body, which contains extended energy.

Pelvic floor exercises (for women)
- To strengthen vaginal and urethral muscles, especially after childbirth.
- Little girls should be encouraged to expand and contract pelvic muscles whilst urinating, to periodically stop and start the flow of urine midstream.
- Lie, sit or stand with legs crossed.
  Imagine the pelvic floor muscles between the legs to be the platform of a lift.
  Contract these muscles to bring them up to an imaginary first floor level and hold. Keep breathing!
  After a while contract the muscles further to the imaginary second floor and hold. Keep breathing!
  Repeat once or twice more.

Regular exercises
- Games are fun and are to be enjoyed!
- Life is a co-operation, not a competition!
- Pursue pleasurable activities that are satisfying.

- Exercising in pools (heated or otherwise!), spas or Jacuzzis is tremendous, especially for the disabled.
- Listen to the body and its needs.
- Sport that is enjoyed is beneficial, sport that is not is detrimental!
- Pressure can cause a variety of sports injuries!

Alexander Technique
- Realigns the body into its natural poise so that energies and life forces can flow freely throughout the whole.
- Society of Teachers of the Alexander Technique, 20 London House, 226 Fulham Road, London SW10 9EL. 071-351 0828.

Osteopathy
- Manipulation of the bone to realign the body.
- General Council and Register of Osteopaths, 56 London Street, Reading, Berkshire RG1 4SQ. 0734 576 585.

Chiropractic treatments
- Bone manipulation for realignment of the body.
- British Chiropractic Association, 29 Whitely Street, Reading, Berkshire RGG 0EG. 0734 757 557.

Homoeopathic remedies
- For rapid relief of acute symptoms between treatments if professional assistance or reflexology massage is not immediately available.
- Seek knowledgeable advice as to actual potencies and dosages.
- Feel at ease about taking natural remedies. If taken sensibly and as directed they are very valuable aids.
- The British Homoeopathic Association, Basildon Court, 27a Devonshire Street, London W1N 1RJ. 071-935 2163.

Acupuncture
- Relieves congested energy flows through the insertion of needles into specific meridian points.
- British Acupuncture Association, 34 Alderney Street, London SW1V 4EU. 071-834 1012.

Crystal Healing
- The value of crystals in healing has been known for centuries.
- A more intense light force is directed through them into the physical and subtle bodies to eliminate negative vibrations.
- Rose quartz held during the massage allows for unconditional love.
- A crystal torch is excellent for balancing the endocrine gland reflexes.

Cutting the bonds (chakras)
- To set others free, with unconditional love and understanding, after a death or at the end of a relationship.
- To release the self from others who appear threatening, demanding or unreasonable.
- This technique can be done at any time, or during meditation.
- Visualise the person concerned, smiling and standing in front of you with all the energy centres between the two of you connected with appropriately coloured ribbons.
- Lovingly, in your mind, cut each ribbon, starting with the red one at the base. See one red end recoil gently back to the other person, and the other red end to the self. Seal the ends in a pink cloud of love. Repeat with the orange ribbon and so on, until all ribbons have been severed. See the person concerned disappear in a pink cloud of love. Do this until feeling completely free and at ease with the self.

Bach flower remedies
- These remedies deal with personality and moods rather than physical symptoms, by easing disharmony at deeper levels.
- They are totally safe with no harmful side effects.
- By identifying their own feelings, recipients should choose the most appropriate remedies for them at a specific moment in time.
- Rescue Remedy, a composite of five remedies, is excellent for panic, hysteria, shock and even unconsciousness. Made up of Star of Bethlehem, Rock Rose, Impatiens, Cherry Plum and Clematis, it is the most useful in any traumatic or emergency situation.

See Appendix 1 for information on each of the remedies.

Music therapy
- Recognises that all atoms, including those making up cells and organs, continually vibrate sending out energies.
- As frequencies change, molecules break apart and re-arrange themselves.
- Each vibrating atom emits an individual sound, so when all bodily parts combine the body has its own characteristic sound.
- Reflexology, with music therapy, reorganises the combination of sounds to produce inner harmony.
- Through healing, the note is restored to its original purity and health is re-established.

Colour therapy
- The energy in the body requires replenishment from the sun's energy in its pure form to remain vibrant and healthy.
- Imbalances occur when one or more colours are not vibrating to their full capacity in specific parts of the body.
- Reflexology opens the body to receive the full spectrum of colour for balance to be re-established.
- If a specific colour is visualised whilst massaging a particular part of the feet, the healing process can be magnified and astounding results accomplished.
- Certain sounds and foods contain colour which, when used in conjunction with reflexology, can be used advantageously to enhance healing.

See Appendix 2 for further information on reflexology and colour therapy.

General tips
- Take pride in personal appearance and choose cheerful, comfortable clothing and footwear. To look good is to feel good!
- Go barefoot as often as possible, particularly over sand, pebbles and uneven surfaces.
- Make space for the self. Have regular facials, pedicures, manicures, etc.

- Create a balance in all aspects of life.
- Enjoy life to the full and live for the here and now.

Footnote: *This section provides food for thought for complete health:*

We are what we think! No one is a threat unless allowed to be. No reason is required to feel good. It is a decision based on the fact that life is for living, not just existing!

Any reference to 'universal power', 'universal strength', 'universal knowledge' and so on refers to the superconscious energy, known as God, the Higher Self, Buddha, etc. This universal energy is a source of inspiration and strength available for everyone regardless of religion, culture, education, skin colour or personality. For this reason, 'universal' is written with a small 'u' to make it more attainable. To tap this valuable life-force, all that is required is an unconditional, heartfelt invitation!

*g*ENERAL GUIDE TO MASSAGE AND *m*ANIPULATION OF REFLEXES

- Both recipient and administrator need to remove shoes and socks/stockings!
- Recipient to lie comfortably either on a reclining chair or on a bed with one pillow under the head and as many pillows as required under the knees and lower legs.
- No effort is required to give a reflexology massage! The therapist should feel energised afterwards.
- Relax and allow the fingers and thumbs to move intuitively. If it feels good then it will be beneficial.
- Massage both feet together whenever possible, otherwise **always** start on the **right** foot and finish on the **left** foot. The **right** foot reflects **past** emotions that need to be released to make way for personal growth and development in the **present/future** aspect of the **left** foot. Until recently it was believed that it was better to massage the receptive and receiving **left** foot first and then the outgoing and giving **right** foot. Although this practice is still acceptable, even better results can be achieved with the new improved technique.
- Before commencing both recipient and administrator should take in three deep breaths for initial relaxation.
- Start by stroking the feet towards you to relax the recipient. This is the only time the movement is away from the recipient.
- Then place the tips of all fingers on tips of little toes. Rest them there for a while. The tingling sensation is the vibration from the exchange of universal energy. Then rest the tips of both third fingers on the tips of the big toes for as long as is felt necessary.
- If in doubt, or if the recipient panics for any reason, immediately pacify through the solar plexus reflexes then, when calm, return to the massage.
- Most people feel totally rejuvenated and extremely relaxed after reflexology. Occasionally, however, symptoms may

intensify as the body eliminates toxic substances. Although possibly disturbing, this is a good sign and indicates that a shift towards health has occurred.
- Provided reflexology is sensitively applied, there are **no harmful side effects**.
- Reflexology provides the recipient with the opportunity to feel better. They can decide to take as much or as little from the massage to meet their own individual needs.

THE MASSAGE TECHNIQUE

The four main movements are:

Caterpillar movement
'Walk' thumbs forwards with the tip of the thumb and the ball of the thumb alternately, soothing the skin's surface.

Rotation massage
Gently place the thumb or finger on the reflex and rotate lightly, either directly on or just above the skin.

Milking movement
Using both thumbs, gently but firmly alternately stroke the skin as though squeezing a tube of toothpaste.

Feathering movement
Use thumb over thumb, or finger over finger to 'feather' stroke the skin's surface in a soothing, rhythmic manner.

The effect of the massage movements

- The **caterpillar** and **rotation** massages create space for physical healing by relieving aches, pain and physical discomfort.
- The **milking** movement calms emotional turmoil and makes space to think straight.
- The **feathering** movement soothes the soul and allows for personal growth and development.

*ℕ*ERVOUS SYSTEM

Definition

Nerves convey conscious, subconscious, unconscious and sensory impulses between the brain and all bodily cells, to evoke decisions and emotions which physically, intellectually and spiritually change the state of mind, body and soul.

Emotional aspect

We are what we think.

Reflexes

In health and dis-ease, the central nervous system reflexes are always massaged first to balance perceptions and encourage the appropriate physical, emotional and spiritual responses. Peripheral nerves infiltrate the whole body so reflexes are reflected throughout both feet.

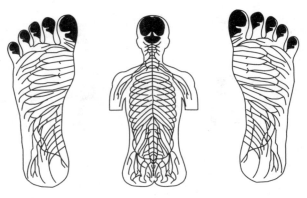

Nervous system

Brain reflexes are found on the pads and nails of all toes, and are massaged to ease tense thoughts, open the mind and relax taut nerves for overall ease. Visualise purple/violet.

Tips of toe pads: Cerebral reflexes for clarity of thought.
Centres of toe pads: Secondary access to hypothalamus and midbrain reflexes for subconscious emotional and physical control and co-ordination.
Base of toe pads: Cervical reflexes for flexibility.

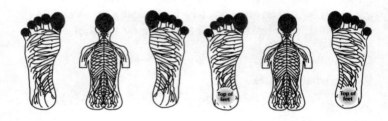

Anterior brain reflexes: Soles   Posterior brain reflexes:Tops

Midbrain reflexes found along the inner edge of the big toes from the tips to the joint bones, are massaged to naturalise cardiac and respiratory functioning as well as muscular co-ordination. Visualise purple/indigo.

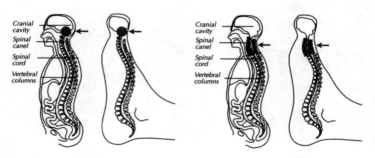

Midbrain reflexes   Cervical or neck reflexes

Cervical or neck reflexes found along the inner edge of the big toes, from the joints to the bases, are massaged for flexibility and adaptability. Visualise turquoise/blue.

Upper spinal (upper back) reflexes found on the inside edges of both feet, from the bases of the big toes to halfway along the bony ridge are massaged for emotional support and to create space for the self. Visualise green.

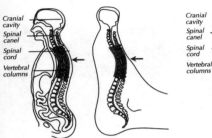

Upper spine reflexes

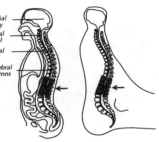

Middle spine reflexes

Middle spinal (middle back) reflexes found on the central portion of the bony ridge on the inner aspects of both feet, are massaged to ease thoughts, feelings and activities. Visualise yellow.

Lower spinal (lower back) reflexes stretch from the centre of the bony ridge to the inner ankle-bone, and are massaged for personal security and a firm foundation from which to grow and develop. Massage the inner ankle-bone well for these reflexes. Visualise orange and red.

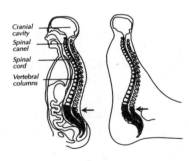

Lower spine reflexes

Solar plexus reflexes found in the hollows immediately below the hard balls in the centre of both feet, are massaged for inner peace, strength and confidence. Lightly place both thumbs on the hollows, with the third fingers resting on the tops of the feet, immediately opposite thumbs. Gradually apply gentle pressure

17

with the thumbs until a slight resistance is felt. Rest the thumbs and hold for a while. Slowly release the pressure, pausing every few seconds to allow the free exchange of energies. Eventually hover the thumbs over the reflexes.

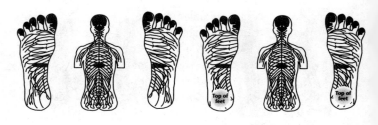

Solar plexus reflexes   *Solar plexus reflexes*

Metamorphic Technique
Place the third fingers on the tips of the big toes. Allow a free flow of energy to establish, then simultaneously run the fingers lightly down the length of both spinal reflexes, to the inner ankle-bones. Repeat several times. This movement helps the subconscious mind to release deeply buried fears and anxieties, suppressed since the time of conception.
The tips of toes: represent the time of conception.
The spinal reflexes: reflect the time in the womb.
The inner ankles: represent the time of birth.

Natural reflexes
All toes reflect brain tissue and perceptions of the mind, with each toe representing a specific aspect of those thoughts:

Big toe(s):	Reflect intuitive perceptions and ideas and are related to the central nervous system. They vibrate to purple, indigo and violet, and are etherical in nature.
Second toe(s):	Reflect thoughts regarding expressions and feelings of unconditional love and self-worth, and are related to the shoulders, upper back, respiratory system, chest, upper arms and legs.

They vibrate to turquoise, blue and green and have an element of air.

Third toe(s): Reflect energetic thoughts regarding activities, self-survival and control and are related to the liver, stomach, spleen, pancreas, middle back, elbows and knees. They vibrate to yellow and contain the element fire.

Fourth toe(s): Reflect thoughts regarding communication, relationships and pleasure, and are related to all circulatory and eliminatory systems, as well as the intestines, lower back, lower arms and legs. They vibrate to orange and have water properties.

Little toe(s): Reflect expansive thoughts regarding mobility, security and possessions and are related to the skeletal and muscular systems, as well as the pelvis, genital organs, base of spine, hands and feet. They vibrate to red and contain the element, earth.

Other suggestions

For a healthy nervous disposition.

- Daily relaxation for clarity of thought.
- Eat wholesome natural foods to feed the mind and nourish the nerves.
- Drink plenty of purified water to flush through toxic substances.
- Stimulate both the logical and creative aspects of mind through work and recreation activities.
- Exercise the brain with thought-provoking, creative ideas.
- Keep an open mind and be forever curious.
- Stretch the toes to stretch the imagination.
- Aromatherapy essential oils:
  Camomile German – to relax the nerves; frankincense – for physical, emotional and mental stimulation; rosemary – to open the mind and intuitional abilities.
- Bach flower remedies for inner peace and understanding.

NERVOUS DISORDERS

Definition

Interference with the natural reception, transmission and/or interpretation of nerve impulses between the brain and the rest of the body, due to tension, swellings or infection.

Emotional aspect

Anxiety distorts thinking and relays confused, conflicting messages to other body parts. There is a fear of being out of control and not coping.

Reflexes

- Central nervous system reflexes, especially the brain reflexes, to reduce intracranial pressure, to ease intense headaches and to make space for the development and growth of new brain cells. The cervical reflexes to release the neck from the grips of tension and the solar plexus reflexes for personal control.
- Endocrine system reflexes, particularly the pituitary, pineal, thymus and adrenal gland reflexes, for emotional control, insight, understanding and inner strength.
- Neck and shoulder reflexes to make space for healing.
- Circulatory reflexes, with emphasis on the heart reflexes, for a natural flow of blood to replenish the supply of essential nutrients.
- Digestive tract reflexes, concentrating on the oesophageal and stomach reflexes, to calm peristalsis and ease the natural expulsion of stomach contents.
- Liver reflexes for the natural elimination of accumulated frustration and fury.
- All bodily reflexes on both feet to reactivate and revitalise the whole.
- Lymphatic and urinary system reflexes for the elimination of all toxic substances to stabilise the internal environment.

For paralysis

Concentrate on the **left brain and face reflexes** on the left toes and the **right spinal reflexes** on the bony ridge of the right foot

or *right side paralysis*. Vice versa for paralysis of the left side of
the body.
For **paralysis of movement**, concentrate on the **lower**
(underneath) aspects of the spinal reflexes and for **lack of
sensitivity and feeling**, concentrate on **upper** aspects of the
spinal reflexes.

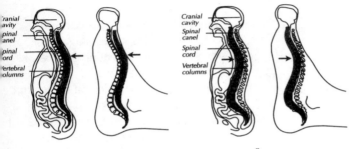

Sensory nerve reflexes   *Motor nerve reflexes*

For head and neck tension and stiffness

Toe pull: Gently but firmly pull individual toes simultaneously,
starting with the little toes. Concentrate on the big toes and
continue to pull for as long as requested. This indirect form of
traction opens the vertebral reflexes and frees trapped nerves,
creating an unrestricted flow of vibrant energy.

Toe rotation or Toe boogie
Gently but firmly rotate each toe individually. Start with the little toe
on the right foot, rotating first anticlockwise, then clockwise, to
loosen stiffness in the neck region. If 'crunching' or 'groaning' is
detected, give extra attention since it indicates accumulated tension!

Achilles stretch
The recipient **must** lie flat and completely straight. Hold the right
heel with the stronger hand, placing the opposite hand in
alignment on top of the foot. Gently but firmly pull with the
underneath hand in one smooth movement. Hold for a moment
then slightly release the pull whilst stretching the foot down with

the top hand. Pull a little further, stretch and then repeat again.

Characteristic Central Nervous System reflexes

Taut	Tips of toe pads:	Irritable, congested thoughts with no space to think.
	Centre of toe pads:	Blocking intuition.
	Base of toe pads:	Determined to move ahead.
	Spinal reflexes:	Rigid, unbending or insecure.
	Solar plexus:	Unrelenting or unresolved emotions.
Flabby	Tips of toe pads:	Giving in and feeling out of control.
	Centre of toe pads:	Given up trying to see other points of view. Indecisive.
	Spinal reflexes:	Feeble support.
	Solar plexus:	Swamped by emotion.
Hard skin		Protects ideas and thoughts.
	Tips of toe pads:	Hides irritability and lack of control.
	Centre of toe pads:	Wearing blinkers. Not wanting to see.
	Base of toe pads:	Determination, obstinacy.
Swellings		Accumulated emotions temporarily inhibit the thought process.
Spinal reflexes	Gap in bones:	A vertebra has been removed or is missing, indicating a lack of support in a specific area.
	Sunken bone:	Support system has collapsed or given in under the strain.
	Gritty feeling:	Either built-up tension or crushed vertebrae.

Other suggestions

- See Nervous System.
- Seek professional guidance.
- Relaxation techniques for peace of mind.
- Massage both feet with aromatherapy oils:

  To lift the spirits: bergamot, clary sage, geranium, jasmine, neroli, orange.

  To calm nerves: camomile, hyssop, lavender, parsley, valerian, vetiver.

  To enhance self-confidence: geranium, jasmine, lavender, rosemary.

  For memory recall: basil, black pepper, cardamon, ginger.

  To refresh the mind: frankincense, grapefruit, lime, rosemary.

  To release nervous tension: camomile.

  To ease headaches and migraines: cyprus, eucalyptus, jasmine, lemongrass, rose, ylang-ylang.

  For clarity of thought: fennel, frankincense, lemon, rose, rosemary.

  For inner peace: fennel, geranium, lavender.

  To alert the senses and for greater impetus: basil, clary sage, lime, neroli, rosemary, sandalwood, ylang-ylang.

  To relieve aches and pains: basil, black pepper, clove.

  To strengthen muscle tone: basil, eucalyptus, lemon.

  To ease spasms: ginger, lavender, marjoram.
- Bach flower remedies for a shift in consciousness, self confidence and peace of mind.
- Services and suggestions for the disabled, forgetful or paralysed:

  MIND, National Association for Mental Health, Granta House, 15–19 Broadway, Stratford, London E15 4BQ.

  MENCAP, The National Society for Mentally Handicapped Children and Adults, 123 Golden Lane, London EC1 0RT.
- Contact a social worker or health visitor to arrange home help and meals-on-wheels.
- Stimulate appetite with small quantities of light, appetising wholesome food containing plenty of roughage.
- Drink plenty of purified fluids.

- Have a book of important details and telephone numbers attached to clothing or bedclothes with string.
- Make the home user-friendly to facilitate mobility and, for those who suffer with convulsions, be extremely wary of loose rugs, electric cables, highly polished floors.
- Have household aids installed, for example, rails throughout the home.
- Use simplified household gadgets, for example, electric can openers, with explicit instructions on a nearby wall.
- Have a shower rather than bath.
- Take pride in your appearance.
- Choose clothing with easily accessible velcro rather than zips and buttons.
- Use a walking stick or aid to keep mobile, and wear sturdy shoes.
- Exercise regularly and invite friends to go for daily walks.
- Do passive exercises initially, becoming more active as muscular control improves, to prevent muscle wastage and to increase locomotion.
- Joints may require supportive splints.
- Keep the mind active by listening to and looking at educational radio and television programmes.
- Keep in contact with friends.
- Find an all-consuming interest.
- Take regular expeditions out of the home.
- Consider occupational therapy and/or therapeutic massages by a trained reflexology therapist and aromatherapist.
- Protect paralysed parts of body from damage and keep them warm, especially if no sensation is felt. Use cushions and pillows to place body and limbs in naturally comfortable positions.
- If speech is affected, provide a pad and pencil to avoid frustration. Also encourage verbal communication.
- Suggest speech therapy if necessary.
- Daily visits.
- Talk about the person's favourite things.
- Express loving feelings towards them.
- Play dolphin, classical and light music.

- Continually encourage by boosting self-esteem and self-worth.
- Give unconditional love and acceptance.
- Provide the tremendous courage and understanding required.

For people with disabilities
- Disabled stickers.
- National key scheme for public toilets.
- Rehabilitation centres.

Royal Association for Disability and Rehabilitation (RADAR), 12 City Forum, 250 City Road, London EC1V 8AF. Tel: 0171 250 3222.

Disability Awareness in Action, 11 Belgrave Road, London SW1V 1RS. Tel: 0171-834 0477

Action on Disability and Development, 23 Lower Keyford, Frome, Somerset BA11 4AP. Tel: 01373 473064

Unit for Disabled Passengers, London Transport, 55 Broadway, London SW1H 0BD. Tel: 0171-918 3312

Footnote: *Change your mind and change your life. Liberate the soul from the bondage of the mind.*

ALZHEIMER'S DISEASE

Definition

Pre-senile dementia due to the death of brain cell tissue with characteristic physical changes.

Emotional aspect

An unsuccessful attempt to control and change everything and everyone, instead of looking to control and change the self.

Reflexes

- As for Nervous Disorders and Insanity.
- Concentrate on all central nervous system reflexes, especially the brain reflexes, to release from the grips of tension and to provide space for the natural development of new brain cell formation.

- Give extra attention to the face, eye, ear, chin, neck and shoulder reflexes for insight and inner strength.

Other suggestions

- Alzheimer's Disease Society, 10 Greencoat Place, London SW1P 1PH. Tel: 0171-306 0606.
- See Nervous Disorders.
- Massage both feet, concentrating on the toes and spinal reflexes, with aromatherapy essential oils to assist in creating a favourable environment for new brain cell formation: basil, black pepper, cardamom, ginger.

Footnote: *Tolerance and kindness to the self creates natural interaction with the universal order of life.*

AMNESIA

Definition

Failed, impaired or loss of memory for certain periods of time. Anterograde amnesia, memory loss for more recent events, or retrograde amnesia for events prior to an accident.

Emotional aspect

The subconscious need to escape emotional conflict and to protect the self against certain fearful events or emotions.

Reflexes

- As for Nervous Disorders.

Other suggestions

- See Nervous Disorders.
- Constantly refer to pleasurable past events, play favourite music and surround with familiar, well-loved objects. Lycopodium – for peace of mind; Bryta Carb. – to recoup mental agility.

Footnote: *Life is a gift, enjoy it!*

ANXIETY

Definition

An emotional state of fear and tension.

Emotional aspect

Uneasy concern about the self due to a lack of confidence, insecurity or extreme fear.

Reflexes

- As for Nervous Disorders.
- Concentrate on all central nervous system reflexes, especially the brain and solar plexus reflexes, to put the mind at ease.
- Neck and shoulder reflexes to unload fears and concerns.

Other suggestions

- See Nervous Disorders.
- Homoeopathic remedies for extra support: Natrum Mur. – to calm nerves; Phosphorus – for reassurance; Pulsatilla – for consistency, emotional understanding and inner strength.

Footnote: *Liberate the soul from the restrictions of the mind.*

APHASIA

See Cerebrovascular Accident

APOPLEXY

See Cerebrovascular Accident

BELL'S PALSY

Definition

One-sided paralysis of the face preventing the eyelid from closing completely. Generally clears up within a few weeks.

Emotional aspect

Disguising true emotions behind a mask of fear and anxiety. Others cannot or will not accept true identity.

Reflexes

- As for Nervous Disorders.
- Central nervous system reflexes to relax the facial nerves and boost self-esteem.
- Concentrate on the facial and eye reflexes for the confidence to project the true self and see life from a brighter point of view.
- Neck and shoulder reflexes to relax the musculature for the free exchange of energies in the head.

Other suggestions

- See Nervous Disorders.
- Look in the mirror and free the self with honest appreciation and unconditional love.
- Protect the open eye, and keep it moist with a few drops of tea-tree oil in a humidifier.
- Massage both feet with aromatherapy essential oils to further enhance the projection of the true personality: frankincense, neroli and rosemary.

BRAIN

Definition

The brain or cerebrum is a collection of nervous tissue that controls all conscious and subconscious activity, linking the physical to the esoterical realms through thought.

Emotional aspect

Thoughts become reality.

Reflexes

- Brain reflexes for clear, inspired thoughts and to elevate the level of consciousness.

Other suggestions

- See for Nervous Disorders.
- Keep an open mind at all times and be forever curious.
- Stretch the toes wide apart to stretch the imagination.

Footnote: *Change your mind to change the quality and nature of your life!*

BRAIN OR CEREBRAL TUMOUR

Definition

Undernourished, swollen, malformed brain cell tissue, deprived of essential nutrients and life forces, due to tension restricting the free exchange of essential life forces and the release of toxic substances.

Emotional aspect

An accumulation of mental tension and pressure which hampers and restricts mobility of thought. Feeling out of control, this further compounds the situation.

Reflexes

- See Nervous Disorders.
- Concentrate on all central nervous system reflexes, particularly the brain reflexes, to relieve headaches, drowsiness and convulsions by reducing intra-cranial pressure, calming nervous irritability, alerting mental faculties and creating space for the formation and development of new, healthy brain cells.
- Give extra attention to the eye reflexes to clear blurred vision by reducing oedema and pressure on the optic nerves.
- Liver reflexes for the subconscious release of accumulated tension and pressure.
- Digestive tract reflexes, especially the oesophageal and stomach reflexes, to counteract nausea and vomiting by calming unnatural peristalsis and by easing the natural expulsion of the stomach contents.

Other suggestions
- See Nervous Disorders.
- Visualise the brain filled with vibrant, healthy cells.

CEREBRAL ABSCESS

Definition
A collection of pus in the cranial cavity believed to spread from a septic disease of the ears, the mastoid cells, the nasal sinuses or due to septic embolism lodging in the brain.

Emotional aspect
Accumulated frustration and anger at not being in control.

Reflexes
- See Nervous Disorders.
- Concentrate on all central nervous system reflexes, particularly the brain reflexes, to ease cranial pressure, to release frustration and to make space for pus to be absorbed by the lymphatic vessels and eliminated from the body.
- Give extra attention to the ear reflexes, if there is an ear infection, to speed up the healing process.
- Circulatory system reflexes for a natural white blood cell content and to replenish brain cells with fresh nutrients.

Other suggestions
- Seek professional guidance in case antibiotics are required.
- See Nervous Disorders.

CEREBRAL ANEURYSM

Spontaneous Subarachnoid Haemorrhage

Definition
Internal bleeding into the subarachnoid space of the brain from a cerebral aneurysm (weakness), or from impact bursting a cerebral blood vessel.

Emotional aspect

Frustration and fury at having decisions and thoughts thwarted.

Reflexes

• See Nervous Disorders.

Other suggestions

• See Nervous Disorders.

Footnote: *Thoughts of joy and unconditional love provide control on all levels.*

CEREBRAL PALSY

Definition

The impaired development of the nervous system, usually due to trauma during childbirth.

Emotional aspect

The physical, emotional and spiritual development of all unborn children is determined by maternal emotions and feelings throughout the pregnancy. Distress, due to emotional disharmony and friction within the mother's environment eg. a car accident or the death of a loved one, can impair development but it is reversible.

Reflexes

Massage the feet of both parents as well as the child.
• See Nervous Disorders.
• Spend time on central nervous system reflexes, particularly the brain, midbrain and spinal reflexes, to create space for the natural development of the nerve tissue and to ease the mind.
• Neck and shoulder reflexes to relax the musculature for the free exchange of life forces between the brain and the body.
• Liver reflexes, for the subconscious release of stored emotions.

- Circulatory system reflexes to provide nourishment for brain cell and nerve fibre development.

Other suggestions

- See Nervous Disorders.
- Support and understand the mother's needs.
- Encourage the child and give unconditional love.
- Relaxation techniques for parents and child, for inner tranquillity.
- Bach flower remedies, especially Rescue Remedy, for strength to cope.

Footnote: *Life is a gift. Allow it full expression.*

CEREBRAL TUMOUR

See Brain Tumour

CEREBRAL VASCULAR ACCIDENT (STROKE)

APOPLEXY

Definition

Sudden paralysis of one side of the body due to intracranial tension which inhibits the natural cerebral blood flow. Due to a lodged blood clot that deprives large numbers of cerebral cells of their essential life forces preventing the natural reception, processing and appropriate responses of nerve impulses. Disturbances occur in the corresponding parts of the body.

Emotional aspect

Feeling deflated and exhausted from resisting the natural life processes. A reluctance to change inhibiting belief systems and principles.

Reflexes

- As for Nervous Disorders.

- Also massage the feet of loved ones.
- Concentrate on central nervous system reflexes, especially the brain and solar plexus reflexes, to relax cerebral tension and for peace of mind.
- Neck and shoulder reflexes for increased flexibility.
- Liver reflexes to release inhibiting belief systems and principles.
- Circulatory system reflexes for the natural absorption of the blood clot and for overall nourishment.

Other suggestions

- See Nervous Disorders.
- Heart Stroke Association, CHSA House, 123–127 Whitecross Street, London EC1Y 8JJ.

COMA

Definition

Complete unconsciousness with absent reflexes due to trauma, infection, poisoning or obstruction.

Emotional aspect

Opting out by initially subconsciously then consciously escaping life's realities.

Reflexes

- Also massage the feet of loved ones.
- Concentrate on all central nervous system reflexes to stimulate conscious and unconscious brain activity and reawaken mental faculties.
- Spend time on all endocrine system reflexes to stimulate emotional response, and for homoeostasis.
- Neck and shoulder reflexes to relax any rigidity for a free exchange of energy.
- Liver reflexes for the subconscious release of total fear.
- Circulatory system reflexes for the natural nourishment of all bodily cells.

- Urinary system reflexes to strengthen sphincters if incontinent or to relax muscular bands if there is retention of urine.
- Lymphatic system reflexes for the ongoing removal of toxic substances.
- All reflexes on both feet to reactivate and alert the mind, body and soul.

Other suggestions

- Seek **immediate** professional guidance.
- Maintain a clear airway.
- See Nervous Disorders.
- Massage the body and both feet frequently with aromatherapy essential oils to stimulate senses further: frankincense, fennel, geranium, jasmine, lavender, rosemary. Also burn in aromalamp.
- Change bodily position regularly.
- Check the body temperature to keep it either warm or cool.
- When consciousness is regained:
  plenty of purified fluids to cleanse the whole;
  passive exercises to strengthen muscles and regain control
- Reassure and support family and friends.
- Bach flower remedies for inner strength, understanding and hope.
- Once conscious, homoeopathic remedies: Arnica – for reassurance; Hypericum – to relieve intracranial pressure and clear the mind; Belladonna – to calm irritability, restlessness and tension; Natrum Sulph. – to ease severe, tearing pain, dizziness and vomiting.

Footnote: *Surround with unconditional love in a secure relaxed environment.*

CONCUSSION

Definition

Injury to the brain due to trauma, causing loss of consciousness. The period and depth depends on the severity of impact.

Emotional aspect

Temporarily subconsciously opting out. Feeling intellectually and emotionally constrained or overwhelmed and unable to cope with present circumstances.

Reflexes

• As for Coma.

Other suggestions

• See Coma.

CONVULSIONS

Fits

Definition

Momentary loss of consciousness with spasmodic contraction of muscles. General illness, trauma or a growth interfere with natural brainwave transmission. A peculiar sensation, taste or smell usually warns of the imminent onset of a major fit.

Emotional aspect

Subconscious resistance to moving with the flow of life.

Reflexes

• See Epilepsy.
• Central nervous system reflexes, particularly the brain, midbrain and spinal reflexes, to naturalise and pacify brainwave activity.
• Concentrate on the ear reflexes, if there is otitis media (middle ear infection), to reduce inflammation.

Other suggestions

• See Epilepsy.

Footnote: *Go with the flow by relinquishing the limitations of human will, ego and intellect. Trust the infinity of universal order.*

CRANIAL NERVE DISEASES

Definition

The interference of cranial function from built-up pressure, infection, an aneurysm or lesion impinging on the nerves within the skull.

Optic nerve involvement: reduces vision and can lead to partial blindness.
Ocular nerve disease: causes drooping eyelids, squints, double vision or unequal pupils.
Trigeminal neuralgia: involves severe jaw, cheek and forehead pain.

Emotional aspect

Built-up frustration, fury and anger at not being in control.

Reflexes

- See Nervous Disorders.
- Concentrate on all central nervous system reflexes, particularly the brain reflexes, to reduce intracranial tension and giddiness, to make space for creative thoughts and to elevate the level of consciousness.
- Give special attention to the face, jaw, eye, ear, neck and shoulder reflexes to release all from the grips of anger.

Other suggestions

- See Nervous Disorders.
- Reduce alcohol intake.

Footnote: *Let go, be yourself and see the beauty of life.*

DEMENTIA PARALYTICA

Definition

Paralysis of the higher brain centres and pyramidal (voluntary) motor tracts with mental deterioration and eventual insanity. Often have ideas of grandeur and delusions.

Emotional aspect

Subconsciously opting out of the real world due to frustration and disappointment with life.

Reflexes

- As for Nervous Disorders.
- Concentrate on all central nervous system reflexes, especially the brain and midbrain reflexes, to release inhibiting thoughts and prevent further deterioration, as well as to strengthen and rebuild the mind.
- Give extra attention to the facial, neck and shoulder reflexes to ease any fine tremor of lips, tongue, or eye especially if there is no reaction to light.

Other suggestions

- See Nervous Disorders.

DEPRESSION

Definition

The lowering of spirits and a feeling of melancholy sadness due to environmental upsets, such as bereavement, disappointment or frustration, or from the personality itself. The latter is known as endogenous depression.

Emotional aspect

Frustration and disappointment at not coping or having control due to losing direction and not understanding the true meaning of life.

Reflexes

- Concentrate on all central nervous system reflexes, especially brain and solar plexus reflexes, to lift the veil of oppression and replace it with insight and inspiration.
- Spend time on all endocrine system reflexes to boost self confidence, emotional strength, inner peace and understanding.

- Neck and shoulder reflexes to release from the grips of anxiety.
- Liver reflexes for the subconscious elimination of pent-up emotions.
- Circulatory, lymphatic and urinary system reflexes to expel old emotions and make way for inner contentment.
- All bodily reflexes to lift the spirits and to inject the whole with enthusiasm.

Other suggestions

- See Nervous Disorders.
- Acknowledge emotions and constructively deal with them.
- Enjoy consuming, pleasurable and rewarding activities and pursuits.
- Mentally cut emotional bonds, especially if the depression is a result of a bereavement or the end of a relationship, to allow the other person to depart in peace.
- Socialise with close friends and break away from the need to isolate the self.
- Take pride in personal appearance.
- Bach flower remedies for emotional strength and support.

DISSEMINATED SCLEROSIS

Definition

Scattered areas of cell degeneration throughout the white matter of the brain and spinal cord with a variety of widespread symptoms. Prolonged remissions of symptoms may occur in the early stages.

Emotional aspect

Scattered thoughts result in the breakdown of communication, confusion and lack of control.

Reflexes

- Concentrate on all central nervous system reflexes, especially the brain and solar plexus reflexes, to restore areas of degeneration, to strengthen lines of communication, to improve co-ordination and for creative patterns of thought.

- Spend time on the eye, neck and shoulder reflexes to calm the optic nerves, to reduce visual disturbance and enhance optimal functioning. Also the throat reflexes to ease tension and improve the peculiar staccato manner of speech.
- Endocrine system reflexes, particularly the pituitary, pineal, thymus and adrenal gland reflexes, for inner strength and understanding.
- Liver reflexes for the subconscious release of pent-up potentially destructive emotions.
- Leg and foot reflexes to increase sensitivity and mobility, especially if partially paralysed, and to improve co-ordination and relieve heaviness.
- Urinary system reflexes, especially the bladder reflexes, to ease urination and relax the muscular sphincters.
- Lymphatic reflexes for the expulsion of wasted, degenerated tissue and emotions.
- All reflexes on both feet to rebuild the natural state of mind, body and soul.

Other suggestions

- See Nervous Disorders.
- Eye exercises to strengthen the optic nerves, especially if vision is disturbed.

Footnote: *Life improves with the realisation that there is not a lack of intelligent people, but courageous ones. Take courage in both hands and believe in the self.*

EPILEPSY

Idiopathic Fits

Definition

A nervous disorder with periodic seizures of the brain cells, depriving them of essential life forces and interfering with the relay of nerve impulses. There is a momentary loss of consciousness, with or without spasmodic convulsions.

Emotional aspect

A temporary loss of control and rejection of life due to spasmodic fear.

Reflexes

- *The specialist **must** be informed of the reflexology treatments so that, with improvement, the drug dosage can be altered accordingly.*
- Concentrate on all central nervous system reflexes, especially the brain and solar plexus reflexes, to ease inner turmoil and conflict, to naturalise nerve impulses and to raise level of consciousness.
- Endocrine system reflexes, particularly the pituitary, pineal, thyroid, thymus and adrenal gland reflexes, to eliminate feelings of persecution, to balance emotions and to create inner peace.
- Neck and shoulder reflexes to ease tension.
- Digestive system reflexes, especially the bowel reflexes to pacify the gastro-intestinal tract.
- Liver reflexes for the subconscious elimination of accumulated turmoil.
- Circulatory, lymphatic and urinary system reflexes to release perceived obstacles for the free flow of life forces.
- All reflexes on both feet for overall well-being.

Other suggestions

- Seek professional guidance.
- See Nervous Disorders.
- British Epilepsy Association, Anstey House, 40 Hanover Square, Leeds LS3 1BE.
- During a fit, place a spatula or similar article between the teeth to prevent the tongue from being bitten, loosen tight clothing, especially around the neck, and make the environment as friendly as possible.
- If fit lasts longer than two minutes seek medical assistance.
- Find suitable 'safe' hobbies and occupations.

Footnote: *Accept the gift of free will with gratitude and choose to create a happier, more tranquil reality.*

FAINTING

Vasovagal Attack

Definition

A temporary loss of consciousness and muscular power, usually of short duration, from a cerebral deprivation of the life forces due to extreme fear or witnessing an unpleasant sight.

Emotional aspect

Temporarily opting out due to fear, lack of courage or loss of nerve. Overcome by the enormity of life. Not coping or feeling in control of circumstances.

Reflexes

• See Nervous Disorders.

Other suggestions

• Loosen tight clothing and allow air to reach the person.
• Put the person's head between their legs or raise their legs above the level of their head.
• Hold aromatherapy essential oils under their nose to speed up the regaining of consciousness: lavender, peppermint, rosemary – also massage both feet, especially the toes, to clear the mind further.
• Encourage the person to sip warm water with lemon and honey.
• Bach flower remedies, particularly Rescue Remedy, for inner strength and reassurance.
• Homoeopathic remedies: Aconite – reduces fear or emotional excitement; Arsenicum – for restlessness, sweating and chilliness; Natrum Mur. – if an emotional or hysterical reaction occurs.

HEADACHES

Definition

Pain and discomfort from throbbing and tension in the head and upper cervical region due to a lack of essential life-forces sustaining the brain cells.

Emotional aspect

Pressurised from too many commitments. Incapable of meeting all obligations.

Reflexes

- See Nervous Disorders.
- Concentrate on the brain, cervical and solar plexus reflexes, to ease the tension and to restore sustenance and order.
- Spend time on:
  facial reflexes, particularly the temple reflexes, to relieve the dull throbbing ache and irritability;
  eye reflexes if sensitive to light;
  neck and shoulder reflexes to release from the grips of tension.
- Toe pull, toe rotation and achilles stretch to ease the pressure on the nerves leaving the spinal cord.

Other suggestions

- To clear the mind further, either inhale the aromatherapy essential oils, or massage both feet, especially the toes, with camomile, lavender, lemongrass, lime, peppermint, rosemary.
- Use ice or heat packs.
- Take in air, preferably fresh!
- Loosen tight clothing.
- Lie down with legs raised above the level of the head.
- Drink lavender or lime flower herb tea.
- Homoeopathic remedies: Arnica – for burning ache in the forehead; Ignatia – to relieve bandlike pressure around the head; Nux Vomica – to ease a splitting headache, dizziness and irritability; Pulsatilla – for periodic throbbing and blinding eye ache.
- Allow others to assist, e.g. ask someone to take and look after the children.

HERPES ZOSTER

See Shingles

HUNTINGTON'S CHOREA

Definition

Involuntary, jerky muscular spasms with a progressive deterioration of the mental faculties.

Emotional aspect

Frustration at having failed to change the world and others.

Reflexes

- Concentrate on all central nervous system reflexes, especially the brain and midbrain reflexes, to create space for new cerebral cell formation, enhanced mental faculties, improved muscular strength and balanced co-ordination.
- Endocrine system reflexes, particularly the pituitary, pineal, thymus and adrenal gland reflexes, for inner understanding and emotional homoeostasis.
- Muscular reflexes especially the neck and shoulder reflexes, for improved tone and greater control.
- Liver reflexes to release accumulated feelings of frustration and defeatism.
- Circulatory and lymphatic system reflexes to flush out self-concern and replace with joyful anticipation.
- All reflexes on both feet to feel in control.

Other suggestions

- See Nervous Disorders.

HYPERACTIVITY

Hyperkinetic Syndrome

Definition

Excessive physical and mental activity. Restless, demanding, impulsive behaviour. Mind flits from one thing to another. Appears to be clumsy with short concentration span. Easily distracted.

Emotional aspect

An overactive mind due to extreme curiosity, but trapped by the physical limitations of life. Escapism from deep fear or feeling pressurised. Often highly intelligent, with thoughts that threaten the tried and tested boundaries of human behaviour, and often beyond the comprehension of others.

Reflexes

- Massage the feet of both parents, as well as the child.
- Concentrate on all central nervous system reflexes, especially the brain reflexes, to pace the mind and allow space for individuality and creativity.
- Endocrine system reflexes, particularly the pituitary, pineal and thymus gland reflexes, for emotional and creative expression in a more controlled manner.
- Muscular system reflexes, specifically the head, neck and shoulder reflexes, to ease tension and hyperactivity.
- Liver reflexes for the natural release of pent-up emotions.
- Circulatory and lymphatic system reflexes to provide mental space within confined physical and emotional boundaries.
- All reflexes on both feet for the harmonious distribution of energy.

Other suggestions

- See Nervous Disorders.
- Hyperactive Children's Support Group, 71 Whyke Lane, Chichester, West Sussex PO19 2LD. Tel: 01903 725182
- Relaxation techniques for parents and child to enhance effective interaction.
- Parental comprehension of the lateral speed at which the child's mind thinks.
- Channel pent-up energy into creative, enjoyable activities that truly express individuality.
- Check to see whether the hyperactivity is caused by any temporary disruption such as moving home, a noisy school environment, the death of a pet or loved one.
- Avoid artificial food colourants and flavourings.

- Bach flower remedies, particularly Rescue Remedy, for inner calm and emotional support.

Footnote: *Inquisitiveness, essential for self-development, needs to be physically paced to accommodate others, but always retain your mental agility.*

HYPERKINETIC SYNDROME

See Hyperactivity

INSANITY

Definition

Mental confusion. Loss of mind control. Appearing mad and senseless. Illogical, incomprehensible behaviour.

Emotional aspect

Subconsciously escaping and withdrawing from the perceived harsh realities of life.

Reflexes

- Concentrate on all central nervous system reflexes, especially the brain reflexes, to centre the self and bring back to reality.
- Endocrine system reflexes, particularly the pituitary, pineal, thyroid, thymus and adrenal gland reflexes, for emotional control and security.
- Neck and shoulder reflexes to create space for the free exchange of energies between the head and body.
- Liver reflexes for the subconscious release of frustration.
- Circulatory, lymphatic and urinary system reflexes to release past fears by unleashing latent contents and creating space for love and joy.
- All reflexes on both feet for the strength to cope and allow everything to fall into perspective.

Other suggestions

- See Nervous Disorders.
- MIND, National Association for Mental Health, 22 Harley Street, London W1N 2ED.
- Understand and cater for individual emotional and physiological needs.
- Provide tremendous love and support.
- Admit to a home if necessary.
- Homoeopathic remedies: Baryta Carb. – for mild confusion.

Footnote: *Life is an opportunity and a challenge. With unconditional love, space and understanding the mind and body instinctively know how to meet it.*

INSOMNIA

Definition

Habitual sleeplessness. Insufficient or unrestorative sleep. Difficulty in drifting off to sleep with long periods of wakeful restlessness, waking up and not going back to sleep or with short periods of interrupted sleep.

Emotional aspect

Overactive mind, overstimulation or overexcitement. Fear, anxiety, guilt or deep concern over unfinished or unsolved aspects, unsettled emotional issues, emotional trauma or physical pain. Sleep is essential for the dreaming process to assist the mind to unravel previous attempts at solving problems and for the body to heal itself. Sleep provides clues to unspoken and unacknowledged fears.

Reflexes

It is best to massage the feet at bedtime so that the person can drift from the alpha state of consciousness into a deep, tranquil sleep.

- All bodily reflexes for overall calm and inner tranquillity.

Other suggestions

- Seek professional guidance.
- Insomnia Self-Help Group, P.O. Box 3087, Chiswick, London W4 4ZP. Tel: 0181-995 8503
- Foot bath with aromatherapy essential oils and also massage both feet, particularly the toe pads, toe necks and spinal reflexes, to further induce deep relaxation of mind, body and soul: camomile Roman, clary sage, lavender, sandalwood, vervain.
- Relaxation techniques to still the mind.
- Avoid watching or listening to the news or violent, disturbing films, particularly at night.
- Use the bedroom for sleeping only – no work, ironing, TV.
- Leave a pad and pencil on the bedside table to jot down ideas and thoughts that come to mind in the alpha state before sleep.
- Exercise daily in the fresh air.
- Create a relaxed, comfortable environment with the correct temperature, and possibly with light music.
- Herbal remedies: camomile tea; lemon balm; vervain herbal tea; a drop of lavender on pillow.
- Place a crystal under the pillow.
- Get up, read or do a jigsaw until ready to sleep.
- Homoeopathic remedies: Chamomilla – for children who are overexcited, in pain or irritable; Cocculus – for overtiredness; Coffea – for restlessness after excessive coffee; Nux Vomica – for fretful sleep with early waking: Passiflora – for an overactive, restless mind; Pulsatilla – for those who fall asleep after midnight and wake early.
- Bach flower remedies, especially Rescue Remedy, to still the mind.

MEMORY LOSS

Definition

Not able to recall or retrieve stored memory.

Emotional aspect

Subconsciously opting out rather than having to face the realities of life.

Reflexes

- As for Nervous Disorders.
- Concentrate on central nervous system reflexes, especially the brain, midbrain and solar plexus reflexes, to calm nerves and for clarity of thought.
- Muscular and skeletal system reflexes, to release from the grips of tension for natural mobility to be re-instated.

Other suggestions

- See Nervous Disorders.
- There needs to be a desire to remember!
- Inhale rosemary or frankincense to clear the mind.
- Jog the memory through observation.
- Stay intellectually alert, motivated and interested in all aspects of life.
- Use mind maps, with patterns to draw out pertinent facts.
- There is no limit as to what the mind can recall.
- Try to remember isolated aspects as part of the whole.
- Use rhymes or mnemonics to remember.
- Avoid alcohol, coffee, drugs, cigarettes.
- Exercise to increase the oxygen supply to the brain.
- Stay calm during anxious moments, e.g. examinations, etc.

MENINGITIS

Definition

Inflammation of one or more of the three meninges, membranes that cover the brain.

Emotional aspect

Subconscious anger at having to cover up inflamed thoughts.

Reflexes

- As for Nervous Disorders.
- Spend time on the brain and cervical reflexes, to reduce inflammation, decrease intracranial pressure and increase neck flexibility.
- Spend time on the eye reflexes and neck reflexes to reduce extreme sensitivity and rigidity.
- Digestive tract, concentrating on the oesophageal, stomach and liver reflexes, to calm irritability, reduce vomiting and release inflamed emotions.
- If there is an initial resistance to touch, hold both feet firmly and lovingly in both hands until a bond and trust is established.

Other suggestions

- See Nervous Disorders.
- Darken the room for photophobia (dislike of light).
- Make the environment friendly in case of convulsions.
- Play dolphin, whale and light classical music.

MIGRAINE HEADACHES

Definition

Tension impinges on the cranial arteries and nerves with episodes of severe headaches, often with nausea, vomiting and visual disturbances.

Emotional aspect

Subconscious resistance to the natural flow of life creates discomfort and pain. Usually affects perfectionists and those with high ideals, who drive themselves beyond the limits and can no longer cope, and yet perceive others to pressurise them.

Reflexes

- As for Nervous Disorders and Headaches.
- Central nervous system reflexes, especially the brain and

solar plexus reflexes, to relax the nerves and release pressure on the brain.
- Concentrate on the eye, neck and shoulder reflexes for relief from pressure, clarity of vision and intuition.

Other suggestions

- See Nervous Disorders.
- British Migraine Association, 178a High Road, Byfleet, Weybridge, Surrey KT14 7ED.
- Stretch all toes open as far as comfortably possible to provide space to think.
- Place ice packs on the forehead and back of head to soothe tension.
- Lie with both feet elevated above the head and concentrate on taking in deep breaths, holding them for as long as possible before letting them go.
- Darken the room and create a peaceful environment.
- Inhale peppermint essence to clear the mind.
- Homoeopathic remedies: Lycopodium – if over right eye, to ease dizziness and nausea; Natrum Mur – to ease throbbing, burning pain; Spigelia – if left-sided, with weakness, fainting and palpitations.

MYALGIC ENCEPHALOMYELITIS (ME)

Yuppie 'flu

Definition

Profound pain and fatigue of muscles, overall weakness and body wasting from inflammation of the brain and spinal cord. Poor concentration, memory lapses, insomnia with hysteria and malingering depression.

Emotional aspect

Subconsciously feeling extremely vulnerable and feeling fearful of being inadequate. Drained of inner resources due to unreasonable expectations of the self. Known as the 'stress' virus.

Reflexes

- As for Nervous Disorders.
- Concentrate on all central nervous system reflexes, particularly the brain and spinal cord reflexes, to focus the mind, calm nerves and trust intuition.
- Endocrine system reflexes, especially the pituitary, thymus and adrenal gland reflexes, for self-confidence, inner-strength and resourcefulness.
- Liver reflexes to release impounded emotions.

Other suggestions

- See Nervous Disorders.
- M.E. Action (Action for M.E.), P.O. Box 1302, Wells, Somerset BA5 2WE.
- Myalgic Encephalomyelitis, Stanhope House, High Street, Stanford le Hope, Essex SS17 0HA.
- Pursue pleasurable, creative activities to boost self-image.
- Listen to the body and rest whenever tired.
- Passive exercises to build up inner strength.
- See Insomnia.

NERVOUS BREAKDOWN

Definition

Drained of nervous energy to the detriment of the whole body.

Emotional aspect

Subconsciously obstructing reasoning and logic along the avenues of communication.

Reflexes

- As for Nervous Disorders.
- Concentrate on all central nervous system reflexes, especially the brain and solar plexus reflexes, to rejuvenate the brain cells for reasonable thought patterns to be re-instated and to open paths of communication.

- Endocrine system reflexes, particularly the pituitary, pineal, thymus and adrenal gland reflexes, for emotional strength and inner resourcefulness.

Other suggestions

- See Nervous Disorders.
- Regularly escape to a new, healthy environment.
- Frequently exercise in the open air.
- Keep busy with creative, rewarding activities.
- Assist the less fortunate.

Footnote: *Re-establish contact with the true self and tap into the fountain of strength and unconditional love within.*

NERVOUSNESS

Definition

Extremely agitated, highly strung, excitable or nervous due to mental unrest and turmoil.

Emotional aspects

Subconscious resistance to the natural flow of life. Little or no faith in the universal order. Extreme fear, anxiety or mistrust.

Reflexes

- As for Nervous Disorders.
- Concentrate on all central nervous system reflexes, especially the solar plexus reflexes, to calm the nerves and raise the level of consciousness.
- Neck and shoulder reflexes to release from the grips of anxiety and allow the free exchange of life-forces.
- Liver reflexes to eliminate extreme agitation.

Other suggestions

- See Nervous Disorders.
- Deep-breathing and relaxation techniques for inner calm.
- Make time and space for self.

- Rebirthing to release suppressed feelings and emotions.
- Self actualisation courses to acknowledge inner strength and talents.

Footnote: *Thoughts create reality. Present thoughts can be altered to create a brighter, more fulfilling future.*

NEURITIS

Neuralgia

Definition

Painful, debilitating inflammation of the nerves, mainly the peripheral nerves. If the arm and leg nerves are affected, there is a loss of motor control causing 'foot-drop' in the lower limbs.

Neuralgia: the sharp, stabbing pain of neuritis.

Emotional aspect

Self-torture due to anguished communication.

Reflexes

- As for Nervous Disorders.
- Concentrate on central nervous system reflexes to ease the mental torture, pain and anxiety and open the channels of communication.
- Liver reflexes for the subconscious release of anguished emotions.
- Muscular reflexes to reduce tenderness.

Other suggestions

- See Nervous Disorders.
- Protect paralysed areas.
- Use a pillow to prop 'foot-drop'.
- Passively massage and move limbs, particularly in warm water.
- Vitamin B supplement to ease nervousness.
- Reduce alcohol and drug intake, if applicable.

PALSY

Definition

Loss of feeling or mobility of any bodily part due to interference of the nerve supply causing utter helplessness of affected area.

Emotional aspect

Extreme panic and fear of life's circumstances paralyses the body, causing a subconscious resistance.

Reflexes

- As for Nervous Disorders.
- Concentrate on central nervous system reflexes especially the brain reflexes on the opposite side to the paralysis and the spinal reflexes on the same side, as well as the solar plexus reflexes, for mobile, sensitive thoughts.
- Endocrine system reflexes, particularly the pituitary, pineal, thymus and adrenal gland reflexes, for emotional control and inner strength.

Other suggestions

- See Nervous Disorders.
- Be as independent as possible.
- Drink plenty of purified fluids to stimulate bodily flow.

PARALYSIS

See Palsy

PARKINSON'S DISEASE

Paralysis Agitans

Definition

Degeneration of basal ganglia brain cells impairing voluntary muscular activity. Uncontrollable twitching of muscles, rigidity of facial expressions, limb tremor, muscular weakness and a peculiar gait.

Emotional aspect

Frustration at not being physically or emotionally in control.
Deeply insecure.

Reflexes

- As for Nervous Disorders.
- Spend time central nervous system reflexes, concentrating on all reflexes, to calm the nerves, centre the mind and raise the level of consciousness.
- Concentrate on facial, neck and shoulder reflexes to release from the grip of fear and anxiety.
- Liver reflexes for the subconscious release of stored emotion.
- Leg reflexes to step ahead with faith and confidence.

Other suggestions

- See Nervous Disorders.
- Parkinson's Disease Society, 22 Upper Woburn Place, London WC1H 0RA.

PETIT MAL

See Epilepsy

POLIOMYELITIS

Polio

Definition

Viral infection causing inflammation of the grey matter of the spinal cord. Possible paralysis and wasting of muscle groups. Polioencephalitis occurs when the inflammation spreads to the midbrain.

Emotional aspect

Paralysing need to subconsciously halt the process of life due to perceived lack of support which threatens individual security.

Reflexes

- As for Nervous Disorders.
- Concentrate on all central nervous system reflexes, particularly the midbrain, cervical and spinal reflexes, to release from the grips of tension for improved tone, flexibility and strength.
- Neck and shoulder reflexes to release the grip on the musculature and for increased flexibility.
- Liver reflexes to eliminate all obstacles.
- Leg and foot reflexes to mobilise paralysed limbs and flaccid muscles.

Other suggestions

- See Nervous Disorders.
- Protect those in the vicinity through immunisation.
- Passive exercises, initially.
- Reassurance that a lost power can be regained.
- Continual encouragement and understanding.

PSYCHIATRIC DISEASE

Definition

Dis-ease of the mind resulting in socially unacceptable behaviour.

Emotional aspect

Subconscious escapism to etherical realms to avoid confronting the physical realities of life. Ideas and beliefs may be too advanced or obscure for modern man at this point in time.

Reflexes

- As for Nervous Disorders and insanity.
- Spend time on central nervous system reflexes, concentrating on all reflexes, to balance the mind and calm the nerves.
- Circulatory, lymphatic and urinary system reflexes for ongoing flow of conscious and subconscious thoughts.

Other suggestions

- See Nervous Disorders.

Footnote: *Blend extraordinary vision with physical reality for the balance of life.*

SCIATICA

Definition

Sharp, stabbing pain down the back of the leg(s), along the sciatic nerve, from the buttock(s) to the ankle(s). Prolapsed vertebrae or a swelling may impinge on the nerve.

Emotional aspect

Confusion and insecurity due to trying continually to please others by conforming to their belief systems and doing that which they expect. The subsequent lack of direction creates a reluctance to move ahead.

Reflexes

- As for Nervous Disorders.
- Concentrate on neck and shoulder reflexes to release from the grips of anxiety.
- Liver reflexes to eliminate confusion and insecure emotions.
- Buttock, leg and foot reflexes to ease the pressure on the sciatic nerve(s) and provide direction to step confidently ahead.

Other suggestions

- See Nervous Disorders.

Footnote: *Move ahead with love, joy and honesty.*

SEIZURES

See Epilepsy

SENILITY

See Alzheimer's Disease

SHINGLES

Definition

Acute skin inflammation with the eventual eruption of small blebs or vesicles which form along the pathway of sensory nerve root ganglion causing excruciating pain. Caused by the chicken-pox virus.

Emotional aspect

Pessimistic views and sensitivity due to fear, tension and anxiety.

Reflexes

- As for Nervous Disorders.
- Spend time on central nervous system reflexes, concentrating on all reflexes, especially the solar plexus reflexes, to calm the nerves and open the mind.
- Concentrate on eye reflexes, if the fifth cranial nerve is involved, to ease the extreme pain and skin eruption. Also to prevent corneal ulceration and promote the growth of healthy new cells.
- Respiratory reflexes, especially if the intercostal nerves are affected, to ease girdle eruption and facilitate the movement of the ribcage.

Other suggestions

- See Nervous Disorders.
- Bio-tissue salts to feed and balance tissues.
- Zinc oxide dusting powder to ease the irritability and pain.
- Care for eyes with drops and regular bathing.
- Homoeopathic remedies: Apis – to relieve burning, stinging pain; Arsenicum – for searing pains that are worse at night; Rhus Tox. – to ease redness and itching of vesicle formation.

Footnote: *Flexibility frees the mind, body and soul from the shackles of self-constraint.*

SPINAL DISORDERS

Definition

The spine physically supports and eases bodily movement through life in an upright position. Interference with this natural function causes disease, pain and disruption.

Emotional aspect

The backbone of life for inner support and resilience. Dis-ease occurs when insecurity shakes and tests the firm foundation.

Upper vertebrae: perceived lack of emotional strength and support especially if carrying heavy emotional burdens or going through a demanding time.

Middle vertebrae: remorse and regret regarding personal activities, which is tucked into the small of the middle back.

Lower back vertebrae: the secure foundation for personal growth and expansion is feeling threatened because there is too great a dependence and concern for material possessions.

Reflexes

- As for Nervous Disorders.
- Concentrate on all central nervous system reflexes, especially the spinal reflexes for natural flexibility and strength.
- Neck and shoulder reflexes to relax the grip on the musculature.
- Lymphatic reflexes to eliminate restraining factors.

Characteristic spinal reflexes

- Firm, flexible instep: solid, reliable support system.
- Fallen or collapsed arch: unable to support the self, e.g. in babies, or a perceived collapsed support system usually during demanding times e.g. break up of a relationship, or death of a loved one.
- Overextended arch: extra resources required to cope with particularly demanding situations, e.g. need to provide extra support after a divorce, death or collapse of a business venture.
- Protruding bone: midway along spinal reflex, affectionately referred to as the 'guilt bump'!

59

Other suggestions

- See Nervous Disorders.
- National Back Pain Association (NBPA), 16 Elmtree Road, Teddington, Middlesex TW11 8ST. Tel: 0181-977 5474/5.
- Association for Spina Bifida and Hydrocephalis (ASBAH), 42 Park Road, Peterborough PE1 2UQ.
- Relaxation technique: Lie on a flat surface with knees bent, breathe in deeply, smile and gently ease the small of the back towards the floor. Do not force the back. Give it time to adjust gradually.
- Check posture at all times and keep the spine straight.
- For more comfort, place the mattress on floor, or on a board.
- Bend knees to pick up heavy objects.
- Alexander technique, body alignment, acupuncture, osteopathy or chiropractic manipulation to assist in realigning the spine.

Footnote: *Support comes from within, physically, emotionally and spiritually.*
Upper back: look to the self for true emotional support.
Middle back: eliminate self-inflicted guilt. Wisdom comes from experience and experience comes from experiencing life.
Lower back: money is an energy. When changes occur on the inside limitless amounts are made available! Owe no one. A generous person who gives unconditionally always prospers!

STROKE

See Cerebrovascular Accident/CVA

VARICELLA

See Shingles

VASOVAGAL ATTACK

See Fainting

$\mathcal{E}$NDOCRINE SYSTEM

ENDOCRINE GLANDS

Definition

Glands without ducts, that are scattered throughout the body. The hypothalamus, below the brain, immediately detects emotional and physical changes and alerts glands to re-establish a state of internal homoeostasis. Hormones are secreted directly into the bloodstream and travel around the body until required by specific target cells, which then absorb and utilise them to balance the whole.

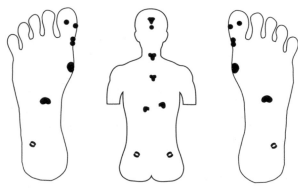

Endocrine system reflexes

Emotional aspect

Harmony of mind, body and soul to facilitate internal and external interaction.

Reflexes

- Always massage the endocrine system reflexes immediately after the central nervous system reflexes because:
  - (i) the hypothalamus determines glandular activity and needs to be balanced first.

(ii) once the central nervous system reflexes and endocrine reflexes have been massaged the clarity of mind, relaxed nerves and emotional stability create sufficient inner peace to reduce dis-ease of the whole substantially.

(iii) the massage of further reflexes throughout the feet soothes individual systems and eases specific congested reflexes.

- Endocrine glands are linked to the energy centres (chakras).
- Before massaging the endocrine gland reflexes, place the tips of the fingers on the tops of the little toes for a few seconds and then the tips of the third fingers on the tops of the big toes for a while, to allow the free exchange of energy to flush through any congestion.
- To massage individual gland reflexes:

  Place both thumbs or third fingers on both reflexes of each gland.

  Gently massage or lightly 'pump' for a few seconds.

  Gradually press gently into both reflexes.

  Hold for a few seconds.

  Release slowly.

  Rest tips of both third fingers lightly on both reflexes for a while, to allow a free exchange of energy (if a strong vibration is felt, relax and allow the energy to be channelled through without resistance).

  Move on to the next pair of reflexes.

Endocrine gland reflexes are massaged in the following order to boost energy and to create inner balance:

Pituitary (Master Gland) reflexes are **always** stimulated first since they control all the other gland reflexes. Their link to the etherical realm through thought and their contact with the higher self, provide ultimate control of the whole. They vibrate to violet.

Pineal Gland reflexes intuitively provide insight and inspiration to ease emotional, physical and spiritual interaction. They vibrate to indigo.

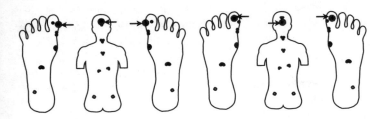

Pituitary reflexes

Pineal reflexes

Thyroid Gland reflexes link the realm of thought with the physical realities of life through the two-way expression of giving and receiving. They vibrate to blue.

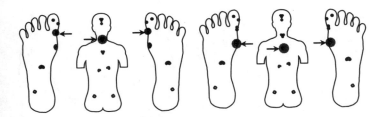

Thyroid reflexes

Thymus reflexes

Thymus Gland reflexes feel unconditional love for life and provide space in which to enjoy it. They vibrate to green.

Pancreatic Gland reflexes provide the energy to respond appropriately to all types of situations and vibrate to yellow.

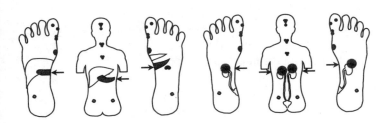

Pancreatic reflexes

Adrenal reflexes

Adrenal Gland reflexes determine those aspects of life that need to be absorbed for self actualisation and those that are no longer of value, easing two-way communication and enhancing relationships. They vibrate to orange.

Sexual Gland reflexes provide basic security for growth, development and mobility and vibrate to red.

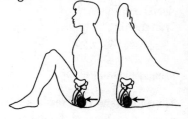

Testes reflexes

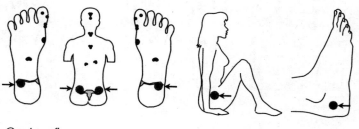

Ovaries reflexes

Ovaries reflexes

JOINING THE ENDOCRINE GLANDS

- Once all reflexes have been balanced join them simultaneously by momentarily resting the third fingers on each pair of reflexes and then running the fingers lightly to link up with the next pair of reflexes.

Begin at the testes/pubic reflexes, stay a while then run the fingers to . . . the prostate/vaginal reflexes, stay a while, then run the fingers over the ankle creases to the outer ankles to . . . the secondary access to ovaries/high stress reflexes, stay a while, then run the fingers under the feet to . . . the ovary reflexes, stay a while, then run the fingers up the centre of the insteps to ... the adrenal gland reflexes, stay a while, then run the fingers to the pancreatic reflexes, stay a while, then run the fingers up the hard balls of the feet to ... the thymus gland reflexes, stay a while, then run the fingers to bases of big toes, then to ... the thyroid gland reflexes, stay a while, then run the fingers to the centres of big toes, then to ... the pineal gland reflexes, stay a while, then run the fingers to the inner joints of the big toes to ... the pituitary gland reflexes, stay a while, then run the fingers to the tips of the big toes, stay a while for a free exchange of energy and then complete the cycle with the Metamorphic technique.

Characteristic reflexes

- Natural reflexes: vibrant and flesh-coloured.
- Swollen reflexes: overactive due to too much going on and excessive emotions.
- Sunken reflexes: underactive due to total exhaustion or giving in to emotions.

Other suggestions

- Trust intuition to be the best guide.
- Enjoy everything you do.
- Life is a balance!

Footnote: *Where there is movement there is life, and where there is life there is hope!*

ENDOCRINE SYSTEM DISORDERS

Definition

Interference with the natural production, secretion, distribution, uptake or utilisation of hormones.

Emotional aspects

Emotional insecurity and uncertainty that tips the balance between health and dis-ease.

Reflexes

The reflexology massage is extremely effective in treating endocrine disorders since it deals with all aspects of imbalance.

For best results concentrate on the following reflexes:
Individual **gland** reflexes for release from the grips of tension thereby creating space for natural hormonal production and secretion.

Circulatory system reflexes to relax surrounding musculature for free flow and adequate blood volume to carry and naturally distribute hormones throughout.

Target cell reflexes (see foot chart for exact site) for the natural uptake of hormones and to create space for expansive utilisation.

One or all aspects may be affected. For example, the gland may be functioning naturally but, due to stress in other parts of the body, distribution is inhibited or tension in the area of the target cells prohibits uptake and utilisation of the hormones.

Other suggestions

- Seek professional guidance.
- Contact a local health visitor and social worker.
- Meals-on-wheels and home help if debilitated.
- Wholesome, natural foods to build up strength.
- Drink plenty of purified fluids.
- Massage both feet with aromatherapy essential oils to further relax the whole musculature: camomile, geranium, lavender, peppermint; for inner peace and joy: geranium, lavender, lemon, rosemary; to accelerate healing: camomile, frankincense, geranium, lavender, lemon; to enhance self-expression: camomile, fennel, frankincense, geranium, lavender, myrrh, rose; to ease discomfort: clary sage, fennel, geranium, rose.
- Passive exercise, particularly in warm water, to build up inner resources.
- Enjoyable, absorbing, creative interest to give meaning back to life.

- Relaxation technique for inner calm.
- Bach flower remedies, especially Rescue Remedy, for hope and inspiration.
- Balance the energy centres through visualisation or meditation, starting with the base centre and finishing in the head.

Footnote: *Live life to the full with endless love, joy and enthusiasm.*

ADDISON'S DISEASE

Definition

Deficiency of the adrenal cortex with muscular weakness, general wasting and extreme debility. Brown pigmentation on the skin and mucous membrane, with darker patches particularly on lips, in mouth and around nipples.

Emotional aspect

Subconscious emotional deprivation of the self from disappointment and frustration with life.

Reflexes

- As for Adrenal Gland Disorders.
- Spend time on the endocrine system reflexes for inner harmony. During a crisis concentrate on the pituitary gland reflexes to reduce the high fever.
- Digestive system reflexes, especially the liver, stomach and colon reflexes, to calm agitated peristalsis. Concentrate on affected areas (see foot chart).

Other suggestions

- Seek professional guidance.
- Contact a local health visitor and social worker.
- Meals-on-wheels and home help if debilitated.
- Wholesome, natural foods to build up strength.

- Drink plenty of purified fluids.
- Massage both feet with aromatherapy essential oils to further relax the whole musculature: camomile, geranium, lavender, peppermint; for inner peace and joy: geranium, lavender, lemon, rosemary; to accelerate healing: camomile, frankincense, geranium, lavender, lemon; to enhance self-expression: camomile, fennel, frankincense, geranium, lavender, myrrh, rose; to ease discomfort: clary sage, fennel, geranium, rose.
- Passive exercise, particularly in warm water, to build up inner resources.
- Enjoyable absorbing, creative interest to give meaning back to life.
- Relaxation technique for inner calm.
- Bach flower remedies, especially Rescue Remedy, for hope and inspiration.

Footnote: *No one can afford the perceived luxury of self-pity when there is an opportunity for a better life!*

ADRENAL GLAND DISORDERS

Definition

Long-term demand on the adrenal glands drains the body of its vitality and energy.

Emotional aspect

The body cannot distinguish between imagined fear in the mind and a genuine threat to survival, so the adrenals remain alert to combat any life-threatening situation – perceived or otherwise.

Reflexes

Adrenal gland reflexes swell noticeably during perceived threatening situations. This is particularly evident in the blind.

- Endocrine reflexes, particularly the pituitary, pineal and adrenal gland reflexes, for emotional strength and security.

- Liver, circulatory, lymphatic and urinary system reflexes to eliminate wasted emotions and make space for the distribution of new, vibrant life-forces.
- All reflexes for courage and belief in the self.

Other suggestions

- Seek Endocrine Disorders.
- Homoeopathic remedies: Natrum Mur. – to calm extreme anxiety; Phosphorus – to reassure and create security; Pulsatilla – for the shy and tearful.

CUSHING'S SYNDROME

Definition

The excessive production and oversecretion of cortisone in the adrenal cortex resulting in an unnatural distribution of fat, abnormal hair growth and atrophy of genital organs. Similar symptoms can occur during steroid therapy.

Emotional aspects

Imbalanced mental activity arising from fear of being crushed by stronger, more threatening forces.

Reflexes

- Central nervous system, particularly the big, third and fourth toes, as well as the solar plexus reflexes, for positive self appraisal.
- Endocrine system reflexes, especially the pituitary, pineal, thymus and adrenal gland reflexes, for emotional strength and inner balance.
- Digestive system reflexes to encourage a balanced distribution of body mass.
- Pancreatic reflexes for the natural functioning and distribution of sugar and to ease diabetes, if present.
- Reproductive system reflexes for an adequate supply of essential nutrients to prevent or naturalise changes of a sexual nature.

- Skeletal system reflexes to strengthen bones.
- Circulatory, lymphatic and urinary system reflexes to eliminate excessive, toxic substances and create space for natural cell formation and development.
- All bodily reflexes for overall harmony.

Other suggestions

- See Endocrine Disorders.
- An operation may be necessary.
- Fill the mind with positive, loving images.
- Consume wholesome, nourishing food to fortify and energise the whole.

GOITRE

Definition

A swelling of the thyroid gland due to overactivity or underactivity.

Simple, non-toxic goitre: simple swelling.

Exophthalmic or toxic goitre: Grave's disease with generalised, diffused enlargement and protruding eyes due to an overactive gland.

Nodular goitre: nodular swelling that is not diffusely enlarged.

Emotional aspect

Subconscious resentment at having little or no time for self-fulfilment and development.

Reflexes

- Central nervous system, especially the solar plexus reflexes, to calm nervous irritability, anxiety and frustration.
- Concentrate on:
    Eye reflexes to reduce exophthalmus and clarify vision.
    Hair reflexes to prevent further hair loss and encourage natural growth.
    Neck and shoulder reflexes to make space for the free exchange of life-forces throughout.

- Endocrine system, particularly the pituitary, pineal, thyroid, thymus and adrenal gland reflexes, to harmonise bodily functions and reduce the size of the thyroid gland.
- Circulatory system reflexes, specifically the heart reflexes, to ease tachycardia.
- Digestive system reflexes, concentrating on the stomach reflexes, to pacify peristalsis and counteract diarrhoea and weight loss.
- Liver reflexes to eliminate stored emotion and fire the whole with natural enthusiasm and energy.
- All bodily reflexes for balanced production, distribution and uptake of thyroxine thereby energising the whole.

Other suggestions

- See Endocrine Disorders.
- Set aside time every day for personal interests.
- Delegate!
- Homoeopathic remedies, but first consult a physician: Iodium – to ease a simple goitre; Natrum mur – to reduce glandular overactivity; Thyroidinum – for exophthalmic, toxic goitre with weight loss, headache, sweating, tremor and agitation.

Footnote: *It is not what is done, but how it is done! Do things because you want to rather than have to!*

HYPERTHYROIDISM

Thyrotoxicosis

Definition

The excessive excretion of thyroxine from an enlarged thyroid gland with restlessness, weight loss despite a large appetite, raised temperature, sleeplessness, increased perspiration as well as rapid respiratory and cardiac rates.

Emotional aspect

Subconsciously fuming at being taken advantage of and then feeling excluded.

Reflexes

- As for Goitre.
- Concentrate on the brain and solar plexus reflexes to centre the self, still the mind and make space for logical thought.
- Liver reflexes to release the build-up of inner emotion.
- All bodily reflexes on both feet to restore health.

Other suggestions

- See Endocrine Disorders.

Footnote: *Centre the self and make time for pleasurable, rewarding pursuits.*

HYPOTHYROIDISM

Definition

A lack of thyroxine due to an underactive thyroid; reduced secretion outpourings; restricted distribution; and/or the inadequate uptake by target cells as a result of tension. A thyroid (gland) that is removed or atrophies causes:

  cretinism in children, with stunted growth and poor mentality.

  myxoedema in adults, with marked swelling of the face and hands, hair loss and mental dullness.

Emotional aspect

Frustration at the lack of opportunity for full personal expression. Resentment for having little or no time for the self, due to complying with the needs and demands of others.

Reflexes

- Central nervous system reflexes, especially the solar plexus reflexes, to alert the mind, improve memory and reduce dull, sluggish mentality.
- Concentrate on the hair, neck and shoulder reflexes to release from the grips of anxiety.
- Endocrine system reflexes, particularly the pituitary, pineal,

thyroid and adrenal gland reflexes for natural hormonal activity, emotional harmony and self-confidence.

- Digestive system reflexes, especially the stomach and liver reflexes, to increase peristaltic activity to avoid or reduce obesity.
- All bodily reflexes on both feet for the natural distribution and utilisation of hormones, especially thyroxine, by stimulating target cell activity.

Other suggestions

- Seek professional advice.
- See Endocrine Disorders.

Footnote: *Create space for the free expression of the self and others!*

OVARY DISORDERS

Definition

The impairment or unnatural functioning of one or both female reproductive glands, which interferes with the production of ova or ovulation.

Ovarian cyst: an unnatural growth, generally filled with fluid. Extreme pain, hormonal imbalance, weight gain and hairiness.

Emotional aspect

Interference with creative abilities.

Ovarian cyst: accumulated frustration and resentment regarding creative aspects.

Reflexes

- Central nervous system reflexes to raise level of conscious creativity.
- Endocrine system reflexes, particularly the pituitary, pineal, thymus and ovary gland reflexes, for inner harmony.
- Liver reflexes for the subconscious release of explosive emotions.

73

- Female reproductive organ reflexes to feel at ease with femininity.
- Circulatory and lymphatic system reflexes, especially the pelvic reflexes, to eliminate obstructions.

Other suggestions

- See Endocrine Disorders.

Footnote: *Provide the creative spark that moves mankind forward.*

PITUITARY GLAND IMBALANCES

Definition

Interference with the production, secretion, distribution or uptake of the hormones secreted by the master gland. An immediate hormonal imbalance occurs throughout.

Acromegaly: the oversecretion of the growth hormone in adults, with no increase in height, but overgrowth of the bone, especially of the jaw, hands and feet, thick, coarse skin and enlarged tongue.

Gigantism: the overactivity of the pituitary gland in children, before the bone epiphyses have united, resulting in excessive weakness and intracranial pressure with vomiting, headaches, blindness and possible coma.

Simmonds' disease: the destruction of the pituitary gland due to a difficult childbirth, tumour or necrosis with retarded development physically and sexually.

Emotional aspect

Lack of emotional control and fear of not coping.

Reflexes

- Central nervous system reflexes, concentrating on all reflexes, to ease intracranial pressure for conscious and unconscious control.

- Endocrine system reflexes, particularly the pituitary, pineal, thymus and adrenal gland reflexes, for emotional control and inner strength.
- Digestive reflexes, especially the liver reflexes, to encourage natural functioning.
- Circulatory, lymphatic and urinary system reflexes to eliminate potential obstacles.
- All reflexes for overall well-being.

Characteristic reflexes

- Swollen reflexes: weighed down with responsibilities and feeling out of control.
- Flat reflexes: worn out from trying to be always in control.

Other suggestions

- See Endocrine Disorders.
- For individual symptoms refer to the specific sections.

Footnote: *Tap into universal energy for intuitive, spiritual control and the perception of miracles.*

TESTICLES DISORDERS

Testes

Definition

Interference with the production of spermatozoa in one or both male glands.

Emotional aspect

Subconscious insecurity with masculine characteristics or gender expectations or due to social pressure and conditioned belief systems.

Reflexes

- Central nervous system reflexes, particularly the big and fifth toes, for self-confidence.

- Endocrine system reflexes, especially the pituitary, pineal, thymus and adrenal gland reflexes, for inner strength and harmony.
- Liver reflexes for the subconscious release of built-up frustration.
- Male reproductive system reflexes, concentrating on the testicle reflexes, to release from the grip of anxiety and fear.
- Circulatory, lymphatic and urinary system reflexes for the free exchange of life-forces.

Other suggestions

- See Endocrine Disorders.
- Massage both feet, especially the toes, heels and ankles, with aromatherapy essential oils to heighten sexuality further: jasmine, neroli, patchouli, rose, rosewood, sandalwood, vetiver.
- Wear loose pants and trousers, especially during leisure periods, so that the testicles can dangle in the cooler temperatures required for spermatozoa production.
- Keep water temperature of baths and showers cool.
- Avoid smoking and drinking excessive amounts of alcohol for healthy spermatozoa.
- Wholesome natural food intake for the natural production of vibrant spermatozoa.

Footnote: *The masculine energy balances universal order and is essential for the survival of mankind.*

THYMUS GLAND

Definition

A ductless gland, situated over the breastbone, below the base of the neck. It is large in early life, but shrivels during childhood until it seems to disappear around adolescence and reappear later in life. However, it remains active throughout life and converts white blood cells into killer T-cells to combat any foreign substances in the body. Gorillas and warriors beat their chests prior to battle to stimulate the natural defences of the body for immediate healing in the event of injury.

Emotional aspect

Keeps the body strong and free of foreign substances. As the seat of the soul, it is extremely vulnerable to any form of abuse. During an emotional onslaught, the hand is often placed over the thymus as a subconscious form of self-protection.

Reflexes

- Stimulation of the thymus reflexes strengthens and reassures the soul of universal support, unconditional love and understanding. Vibrates to green and pink.
- Concentrate on the thymus reflexes on the young, elderly, sick and those suffering with AIDS and myalgic encephalomyelitis.

Characteristic reflexes

- Hard skin over the reflex: indicates a subconscious need to protect the self against verbal, emotional or physical abuse.
- Hollow reflexes: the natural state in adults but if in children, the elderly or if particularly sunken, it indicates eating away at the self.
- Swollen reflexes: fighting to maintain individuality.

Other suggestions

- Beat chest, on either side of breastbone, every day, to boost natural immunity and to provide inner strength and confidence to be the true self.

THYROID GLAND

See Goitre, Hyperthyroidism and Hypothyroidism

Definition

A ductless gland consisting of two lobes at the front of the trachea, which produces and secretes thyroxine for body metabolism.

Emotional aspect

Makes space for self expression. Imbalances occur with resentment at always having to be there and do things for others.

Reflexes

- Stimulation of the thyroid gland reflexes provides the balance in life.

Characteristic reflexes

- Natural reflexes: gritty, sensitive swellings.
- Swollen reflexes: indicates overactivity or accumulated resentful emotions.
- Sunken reflexes: indicates underactivity or total exhaustion from being at the beck and call of others.
- Taut or hard reflexes: may be scar tissue if a thyroidectomy (removal of the thyroid gland) has been performed, or indicates an emotional resistance.
- Hard skin over reflexes: subconscious need to protect own time and space.
- Flaking skin over reflexes: irritability at not being allowed to be an individual.

Other suggestions

- Delegate tasks to other family members and colleagues to leave more time for the self.
- Instead of feeling compelled to have to do things grudgingly, do them because you **want** to. A change of approach makes all the difference!
- Make space for the self and others.

Footnote: *Be kind and considerate to the self by expressing the true self to the benefit of mankind.*

hEAD, NECK AND SENSORY ORGANS

HEAD AND FACE

Definition

The head is the exchange centre for all vital energies. The face is the most exposed part of the head which is presented to the world.

Emotional aspect

Through conscious, subconscious, unconscious and intuitive activity, appropriate internal and external interaction and communication is motivated in a comprehensive, decisive manner. Changing expressions of the face's countenance outwardly portray emotions and project inner feelings based on reactions to present and past situations. The expressions of life's journey are mapped out and make their impression on the face, although true emotions are often masked by putting on a front. Every experience leaves its mark temporarily or permanently.

Reflexes

Head reflexes, found on all toes, with the big toes being the main reflexes. Massage of these reflexes eases interaction between the etherical world of thought and the physical reality of ideas being put into action. They vibrate to purple/turquoise.

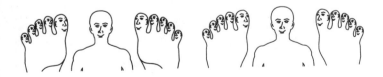

Face and Head reflexes   Head reflexes

Face reflexes found on the balls of all toes. Massage to nurture and relax countenance.
They vibrate to purple/turquoise.

Hair reflexes found on the tips and tops of all toes, are massaged to provide natural protection from outside forces.
They vibrate to purple/turquoise.

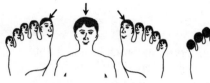 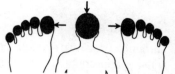

Hair reflexes (Primary - soles)   *Hair reflexes (secondary - tops)*

Temple reflexes found on the tips of all the toes, are massaged to encourage the free exchange of energies and to create space for the thought process.
They vibrate to purple/turquoise.

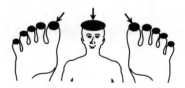 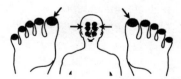

Temple reflexes   *Sinus reflexes*

Sinus reflexes found on the tips of all the toes, are massaged to provide space for conscious thought and space to play around with ideas.
They vibrate to purple/turquoise.

Eye reflexes found at the centres of the toe pads, with the main reflexes on the big toes, are massaged to enhance vision and insight.
They vibrate to purple/turquoise.

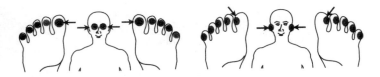

Eye reflexes   Ear reflexes

Ear reflexes found on the joints on either side of each toe, with the outer ear reflexes on the little toes and the inner ear reflexes on the big toes, are massaged for natural balance and the appropriate interpretation of and reaction to sounds.
They vibrate to purple/turquoise.
Lace fingers between toes and gently squeeze them against toe joints to stimulate all ear reflexes at the same time.

Nose reflexes found in the inner aspect of all joints, particularly the big toes, are massaged to heighten the senses and self recognition. They vibrate to purple/turquoise.

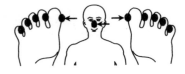

Nose reflexes

Cheek reflexes found on the outer aspect of the joints on each toe, especially the big toes, are massaged to provide encouragement to face the world with confidence.
They vibrate to purple/turquoise.

81

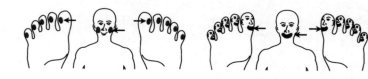

Cheek reflexes

Mouth reflexes

Mouth reflexes found in the inner aspect of all toe pads towards the base, are massaged to ease the exchange of expressions between the inner and outer environments. They vibrate to purple/turquoise.

Gum reflexes – as for mouth reflexes, are massaged to secure decisions.
They vibrate to purple/turquoise.

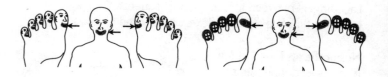

Gum reflexes

Teeth reflexes

Teeth reflexes – as for mouth reflexes, are massaged for firm decisions.
They vibrate to purple/turquoise.

Tongue reflexes – as for mouth reflexes, are massaged for the ability to savour life's experiences with ease and understanding. They vibrate to purple/turquoise.

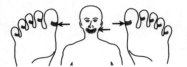

Tongue reflexes

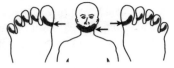

Jaw reflexes

Jaw and Chin reflexes found along the bases of all toe pads, are massaged for mobility of expression.
They vibrate to turquoise/blue.

Neck and Throat reflexes found on the necks of all toes, especially the big toes, are massaged to ease the exchange and interaction of true expressions between the physical and etherical realm.
They vibrate to turquoise/blue.

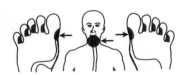

Throat reflexes

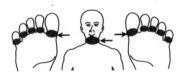

Neck reflexes

Characteristic reflexes

- Hard skin over mouth reflexes: from having to keep the mouth shut!
- Hard skin over the nose reflexes: to prevent the nose from being knocked out of joint.

- Hard skin over sinus reflexes: hiding irritability.
  if covered with flaking skin: irritated at hiding irritability.
- Hard skin over jaw reflexes: from gritting the teeth in determination or from being obstinate!
- Also see the eye and ear reflexes.

Other suggestions

- Frequent herbal and cleansing facials. To look good is to feel good.
- Skin care through moisturisers and protection.
- Wear a hat when in direct sunlight.
- Enjoy life to the full to avoid deep impressions and marks of emotional turmoils being engraved on the countenance.

ADENOID GLANDS – SWOLLEN

Definition

Mass of spongy tissue at the top of the throat that swells and interferes with the breathing. More common during childhood.

Emotional aspect

A lump in the throat. Build-up of emotional congestion and stifled creativity.

Reflexes

Massage the feet of both parents as well as the child.

- Concentrate on the central nervous reflexes, especially the solar plexus reflexes, to alter perceptions and boost self-worth.
- Concentrate on the neck and shoulder reflexes to ease lumps of emotion.

Other suggestions

- Seek professional guidance if severe.
- Inhale aromatherapy essential oils and use to massage the feet, particularly along the necks of the toes, to further ease congestion: eucalyptus, lavender, tea-tree.

- Sip warm water, lemon and honey.

Footnote: Attract only loving thoughts through thinking and emitting loving thoughts.

BLEEDING GUMS

Definition

Bleeding from the fleshy jaws in which teeth are embedded.

Emotional aspect

Sadness concerning decisions made to please others rather than the self.

Reflexes

- As for Mouth Disorders.
- Concentrate on facial, neck and shoulder reflexes for a free flow of energy to the jaw.

Other suggestions

- See Mouth Disorders.

BLINDNESS

Definition

Permanent or temporary deprivation of sight.

Emotional aspect

Subconsciously turning a blind eye. Fear of seeing and not coping with an exceptionally emotional and traumatic situation.

Reflexes

- As for the eye reflexes.
- Concentrate on the brain, the eye and the shoulder reflexes to stimulate optic nerves and open the mind for enhanced insight and nurture the optic area.

- The adrenal reflexes which are generally swollen due to extreme vulnerability and the innate need to be continually on the defensive.
- Liver reflexes for the subconscious relief of the blinding terror.

Other suggestions

- Royal National College for the Blind, College Road, Hereford HR1 1EB. Tel: 01432 265725
- Seek professional guidance.
- Inform a local health visitor and social worker.
- Massage both feet, especially the toe pads, with aromatherapy essential oils to further increase inner calm: frankincense, juniper, lavender, rosemary.
- Be as independent as possible.
- See Nervous Disorders.
- Live in environment friendly surroundings with everything at hand.
- Label all containers in braille.
- Inner visualisation to stimulate senses. Easier for the previously sighted.
- Investigate and take full advantage of libraries for the blind, tape recorders and other useful gadgets.
- Learn reflexology, massage or other forms of healing through a professional training school. Some of the best therapists are blind.
- Take pride in personal appearance.
- Bach flower remedies, particularly Rescue Remedy, for reassurance and inner strength to cope.

CATARACTS

See Eye Disorders

COLD SORE

See Skin

CONJUNCTIVITIS

See Eye Disorders

DEAFNESS

Definition
Total or partial loss of hearing.

Emotional aspect
Turning a 'deaf ear' to avoid internal conflict or to shut out others' opinions. Negative cluttered thoughts block the hearing process particularly during emotional distress, when meaning and interpretation of words becomes distorted or amplified, further aggravating the trauma.

Reflexes
- As for Ears.
- Concentrate on the ear reflexes to stimulate the auditory nerves and create a healthy environment for new cell formation to re-establish natural functioning, and the sinus reflexes to clear the head.

Other suggestions
- Seek professional guidance.
- Learn sign language and lip-reading.
- Massage both feet, particularly the sides of the toes, with aromatherapy essential oils to enhance inner peace and tranquillity: camomile, geranium, jasmine, neroli, lemon, rose, rosemary.
- Be as independent as possible.
- Touch others as they speak to feel the vibration of their voice, which will enhance understanding.
- Homoeopathic remedies: Iodine – for temporary catarrhal deafness; Phosphorus – to ease anxiety when too many noises cause confusion; Pulsatilla – for roaring pains and possible discharge.
- Bach flower remedies for inner strength and understanding.

EARS

Definition

Organs of hearing and balance that inherently receive sounds from outside the body to orientate the mind towards surrounding vibrations. Balance provides a sense of proportion during motion.

Emotional aspect

Facilitate the capacity to hear, interpret and absorb noise vibrations by tapping into the vast and intriguing world of sound. The brain's interpretation of these sounds determines actions and reactions.

Reflexes

- Massage the ear reflexes, for natural balance and the appropriate interpretation and reaction to sounds.
- Central nervous system, especially the brain reflexes, to stimulate the auditory nerves, calm the mind, relieve pain and facilitate the relay of sound waves for the appropriate interpretation and reaction to sounds.
- Concentrate on: the ear and sinus reflexes to release from the grip of fear and anxiety to ease reception and transmission of sound waves. Lace fingers between toes and gently squeeze against the toe joints to stimulate all ear reflexes simultaneously, and the neck, jaw and shoulder reflexes to relax musculature for a free flow of blood to the ears.

Other suggestions

- Exercise ears by listening, hearing and understanding everything!
- Many sounds are heard although not all are understood, for example, a foreign language, but still listen to all sounds with wonderment and curiosity.
- Music therapy for the therapeutic value of sounds.

Footnote: *Open your ears to life's vibrations and accept them with unconditional love, appreciation and gratitude.*

EARACHE – OTITIS

External, middle or inner ear infections

Definition

Acute infection and inflammation of the ear from the invasion of irritable foreign microbes. Severe infection of the middle ear, otitis media, can lead to temporary deafness. The build-up of infected cells in the middle ear can inhibit the mobility of the three small bones, preventing the transmission of sound from the external to the inner ears.

Emotional aspect

Vibrations of unpleasant, conscious or subconscious, thoughts disrupt and threaten peace and security within the environment.

Reflexes

- As for Ears.
- Concentrate on the endocrine system reflexes, particularly the pituitary, pineal, thymus and adrenal gland reflexes, to reduce inflammation and for emotional control.
- Liver reflexes to release stored anger and irritation.

Other suggestions

- Seek professional guidance if severe.
- Massage both feet, especially the sides of the toes, with aromatherapy essential oils to assist in expelling toxic substances: camomile, lavender, tea-tree; also warm a teaspoonful of olive oil, put on cotton wool and place in the ear.
- Apply local heat to reduce the pain.
- Homoeopathic remedies: Aconite – to ease the acute onset of pain and fever; Belladonna – to calm throbbing ears accompanied by headache and sore throat. Mercurius – to relieve the sharp, severe pain with pus or blood discharge. Plantago Tincture – use locally if there is no discharge. Sulphur – to ease recurrent earaches with continual discharge.
- Bach flower remedies to release unwanted emotions.

EYES

Definition

Projections of brain tissue that come to the surface to provide two-way communication with the outside world through visual impressions and energy vibrations. They provide a sense of space and proportion. The irises reflect a complete map and pattern of bodily functions.

Emotional aspect

Eyes provide the means to see the whole spectrum of life in an unprejudiced manner. The irises reflect characteristics and emotions of the inner being. The right eye reflects the past and the left, the present/future, whilst colour indicates the chakra level that requires the greatest energy, hence the reason why eyes change colour or differ.

Reflexes

- Massage the eye reflexes for optimum vision.
- The pineal gland secretions rely on the amount of natural daylight entering the eyes.

Characteristic reflexes

- Swollen reflexes: not wanting to see and blocking intuition.
- Flabby and sunken reflexes: disinterested in that which is seen.
- Hard reflexes: resisting the two-way interaction of light vibrations.

Other suggestions

- Close eyes and 'look' directly at the sun to re-energise.
- Eye exercises to strengthen the eyes.
- Place cucumber slices over the eyes to keep refreshed.
- To prevent eye strain check posture, blink and breathe often and take eyes away from the object concerned at frequent intervals.
- See something of interest in all activities.

EYE DISORDERS

Definition

Interference with the reception, reaction or interpretation of light vibrations.

Astigmatism: a defective curvature of the eye causing diffused vision.

Cataracts: dim vision due to the clouding of lens.

Farsightedness: hypermetropia, the eyeball is too short and light converges beyond the retina.

Nearsightedness: myopia, the eyeball is too long and light converges before the retina.

Conjunctivitis: inflammation of the conjunctiva.

Keratitis: inflammation of the cornea.

Glaucoma: poor drainage of the aqueous fluid due to raised intraocular pressure.

Styes: hordeolum, inflammation of sebaceous gland within the eyelashes.

Eye strain: fatigue of visual functions.

Emotional aspect

Turning a blind eye. Putting on blinkers to block out emotionally distressing sights. Preventing insight into seeing truth about the self.

Astigmatism: avoiding focusing on the self. Extreme fear of seeing hurtful emotions that threaten security.

Cataracts: blocking out a bleak, depressing future and foreseeing visions of hopelessness.

Farsightedness: plans ahead by projecting into the future.

Nearsightedness: manifests within two years of an emotionally traumatic experience that creates a deep distrust of seeing ahead.

Keratitis and conjunctivitis: deep anger at that which is being perceived visually.

Stye: viewing life or a person through angry eyes.

Reflexes

- Central nervous system reflexes, especially the brain reflexes, to still the mind, calm the nerves and nourish the optic nerves, allowing light impulses to be interpreted efficiently and creatively.

- Concentrate on: the eye reflexes to enhance visual perception and intuition, and the sinus, jaw, throat and shoulder reflexes to ease congestion.
- Endocrine system reflexes, particularly the pituitary, pineal and adrenal glands, for emotional control and balance. Pineal secretions, controlled by amount of natural light entering the body through the eyes, determine mood swings which directly influence the perceptions and interpretation of light images.
- Respiratory reflexes for the free exchange of essential forces.
- Liver reflexes to remove anger and create a relaxed internal environment allowing the eyes to open without prejudice.
- Circulatory and lymphatic system reflexes for a free flow and exchange of life energies.
- Urinary system reflexes, especially the kidney reflexes, for a stable watery environment.

Other suggestions

- Seek professional guidance.
- Massage both feet, particularly the toe pads and necks, with aromatherapy essential oils for deeper insight and understanding: camomile, fennel, geranium, jasmine, lavender, peppermint.
- Exercise eyes by looking expansively and seeing every detail.
- Homoeopathic remedies:

    Cataracts   Calc. Phos. – to ease misty, diminished, blurred vision; Conium – for light intolerance.

    Eye strain   Calcarea and Ledum – for aching, tired eyes; Euphrasia – to clear blurred vision; Gelsemium – to ease overworked eyes.

    Glaucoma   Aconite – for acute glaucoma; Bryonia – to reduce intraocular pressure; Phosphorus – to diminish pain and limit degeneration.

- Avoid sunglasses because they weaken the eyes by denying them the opportunity to expand and contract naturally to accommodate fluctuations of light.

- See Eyes.
- Remove spectacles and avoid using contact lenses frequently to strengthen the eyes.

Footnote: *See life from every point of view.*

GUM DISORDERS

Definition

Disorders of the firm flesh in which teeth are embedded.

Emotional aspect

Difficulty in coming to terms with decisions. Uncertainty. Not feeling secure or happy about decisions made.

Reflexes

- As Mouth Disorders.
- Concentrate on the mouth, chin, neck and shoulder reflexes especially the big toes, to relax the jaw and renourish gums.

Other suggestions

- See Mouth Disorders.

HAY FEVER

See also Allergies

Definition

Hypersensitivity of the nasal and sinus mucous membranes due to extreme sensitivity causing sneezing, runny blocked nose, acute catarrh, itchy eyes, scratchy throat and possible wheezing.

Emotional aspect

Often perfectionists who expect high standards from themselves and from others. Irritability builds up as expectations are not met and frustration arises from others not being able to do things 'properly'.

Reflexes

- As for Sinusitis.
- Concentrate on the sinus, nose, eye, neck and shoulder reflexes to ease congestion.
- Respiratory system reflexes to expand the chest and ease the interchange of energies.

Other suggestions

- Massage both feet, concentrating on the toe pads and toe necks, with aromatherapy essential oils to further ease the congestion: camomile, eucalyptus, lavender, lemon.
- Also use for inhalations, aromalamps and in the bath.
- Use ioniser to cleanse environmental atmosphere.
- Homoeopathic remedies to further desensitise the whole and for long-term stimulation of immune system. Also: Arsenicum – if worse after midnight; Kali Carb. – relieves severe symptoms; Sabadilla – eases profuse watery discharge.

JAW DISORDERS

Temporomandibular Joint Disorders

TMJ Syndrome

Definition

Two sets of bones that form the mouth's framework, used for chewing and verbal expression. Tension interferes with the natural mobility and utilisation of the joint.

Emotional aspect

'Gritting the teeth' and 'setting the jaw'. Extreme determination, resentment, frustration, obstinacy, anger or revenge.

Reflexes

- Central nervous system reflexes, particularly the solar plexus reflexes, to release nervous tension.
- Concentrate on the facial reflexes, especially the jawline, neck and shoulder reflexes, to relax and restore mobility.

- Endocrine system reflexes, for inner peace.
- Liver, circulatory, lymphatic and urinary system reflexes to eliminate toxic substances and release emotional hurts.

Other suggestions

- See Tooth and Mouth Disorders.

Footnote: *Trust the flow of life to soothe and give direction.*

LARYNGITIS

Definition

Inflamed larynx causing temporary hoarseness or loss of voice.

Emotional aspect

Anger at not being heard. Fear of expressing self for fear of ridicule, shame or lack of self-confidence. Resentful of authority.

Reflexes

- See Throat Disorders.
- Concentrate on the neck, throat and shoulder reflexes to relax the vocal cords and encourage free expression of true feelings.

Other suggestions

- Massage both feet with aromatherapy essential oils, to increase inner tranquillity: camomile, fennel, lavender, lemon, peppermint, thyme. Also use in steam inhalations.
- Eat light, nutritious, wholesome food to fortify the whole.
- Drink plenty of soothing, purified fluids to calm the throat.
- A well-ventilated environment to clear the air.
- Bach flower remedies to boost self-confidence.
- Homoeopathic remedies: Arnica – to ease a painful, swollen larynx, especially if due to shock. Causticum – to relieve hoarseness and dry rawness; Oxalic Acid – for severe cases with painful raw sensation.
- Find an avenue to channel expression creatively, e.g. painting, writing stories, singing.

LOCKJAW

Tetanus

Definition

Tonic spasm of chewing muscles with rigidity and closure of jaws.

Emotional aspect

Subconsciously clenching the teeth in frustration, anger and/or obstinacy from insecurity.

Reflexes

- Concentrate on the face, jaw, neck and shoulder reflexes to release from the vice-like grip of tension.

Other suggestions

- Seek professional guidance.
- Massage both feet with aromatherapy oils, concentrating on the lower part of the toe pads and the toe necks, for further peace and tranquillity: camomile, eucalyptus, ginger, peppermint.
- Bach flower remedies for inner strength and understanding.
- Relaxation techniques to further ease the mind.

LOSS OF BALANCE

Definition

Unsteady due to dizziness or other interference with the natural posture.

Emotional aspect

Excessive emotional turmoil, conflict or confusion.

Reflexes

- As for Earache.
- Concentrate particularly on: the ear reflexes to balance the

inner ear; the jaw, neck and shoulder reflexes to relax the musculature.

Other suggestions

- Massage both feet, especially the sides and the toe pads, with aromatherapy essential oils to enhance balance and inner stability: bergamot, fennel, geranium, ginger, lavender, lemon, rosemary.
- Relaxation techniques for inner peace.
- Vitamin and mineral supplements to fortify the self.
- Bach flower remedies for the balance of life.

MASTOIDITIS

Definition

Inflammation of the mastoid antrum, the cavity in the skull that communicates with the middle ear.

Emotional aspect

Fear, frustration and anger at what is being heard because it creates inner turmoil, conflict or insecurity.

Reflexes

- As for Earache.
- Concentrate on the ear, neck and shoulder reflexes to calm inner turmoil.
- Liver reflexes to release inflamed emotions.

Other suggestions

- See Ear Disorders.

MOUTH DISORDERS

Definition

Interference with functions of chewing or vocal utterances.

Emotional aspects

Inability to express the true self or reluctance to break down new ideas.

Reflexes

- Central nervous system reflexes to open mind and encourage flexibility.
- Concentrate on the facial reflexes, especially the mouth, neck and shoulder reflexes, to release from the grip of rigidity.
- Endocrine system reflexes, especially the pituitary, pineal, thymus and adrenal gland reflexes, for emotional control.
- Digestive system reflexes to enhance nutrition of mind, body and soul.
- Liver, circulatory, lymphatic and urinary system reflexes to eliminate toxic substances and suppressed emotions.

Other suggestions

- Massage both feet, particularly the toe pads, with aromatherapy essential oils to accelerate the healing process: camomile, geranium, lavender, tea-tree.
- Oral hygiene with regular mouthwashes.
- Raspberry leaf tea gargle.

NEARSIGHTEDNESS

See Eyes

NECK DISORDERS

See also Stiff Neck

Definition

Interference with the head's mobility and flexibility.

Emotional aspect

Single-mindedness. Preventing free exchange of energies between the realm of thought and the physical body.

Reflexes

- Central nervous system reflexes, especially the cervical vertebrae reflexes, to loosen set concepts and open the mind to other options.
- Concentrate on the neck reflexes to increase mobility.
- Endocrine system reflexes, with attention to the pituitary, pineal and adrenal gland reflexes, for emotional and intuitive control.
- Shoulder reflexes to ease the strain.
- Liver reflexes to release accumulated emotions.
- Circulatory, lymphatic and urinary system reflexes, particularly in the neck region, to release the build up of toxic emotions and feelings.
- All reflexes in both feet to release the whole from the grips of rigidity.
- Toe pull and rotation to free tension trapped in the neck region.
- Achilles stretch to expand and extend the whole.
- General manipulation of both feet for overall flexibility.

Other suggestions

- If severe, seek professional guidance.
- Massage both feet with aromatherapy essential oils, concentrating on the necks and bases of the toes, to ease tension further: black pepper, ginger, peppermint, rosemary. Also use to massage neck area.
- For associated headache, massage the neck with three to five drops of peppermint oil dissolved in a teaspoon of vegetable oil.
- Ice-packs in neck and shoulder region, to soothe the area.
- Relaxation techniques for peace of mind.
- Bach flower remedies for inner security.

NOSE DISORDERS

Definition

Interference with the organ of smell and respiration which prevents the natural cleansing and heating of atmospheric air to the body's requirements and inhibits the ability to detect and respond appropriately to environmental aromas.

Nose bleeds: outpouring of blood from the nasal cavity.
Runny nose: constant flow of mucus from the nasal cavity.
Stuffy nose: congested nasal passages.

Emotional aspect

Subconscious belief that personal recognition is threatened.
Difficulty in adapting to changes within the environment.

Nose bleeds: nose knocked out of joint. Deep sadness at perceivably not being acknowledged.
Runny nose: flushing out the old to make space for the new.
Stuffy nose: feeling 'bunged up' and extremely irritable at not acknowledging or accepting self-worth.

Reflexes

- All central nervous system reflexes for self-acknowledgement.
- Concentrate on the nasal, chin, neck and shoulder reflexes to heighten the sense of taste and smell and for personal recognition.
- Endocrine system reflexes to balance emotions.
- Liver reflexes to fire the individual with enthusiasm.
- Lymphatic system reflexes, particularly in the nasal region, to ease congestion by flushing out outdated concepts.
- All reflexes particularly if weakness, fainting, anaemia and pallor are present to strengthen and energise the whole.

Other suggestions

- Seek professional guidance, if severe.
- Inhale lemon or lavender essential aromatherapy oils.
- Use ice packs or pinch bridge of nose to constrict blood vessels and stem the flow of blood.
- See Anaemia and Fainting if applicable.
- Homoeopathic remedies: Arnica – to ease the shock; Belladonna – to relieve cerebral congestion; Hamamelis – use either externally as a tincture or internally as a pill to ease symptoms; Vipera 200 – to arrest haemorrhage.
- Bach flower remedies for self-confidence.

PERITONSILLAR ABSCESS

See Throat Disorders

POST NASAL DRIP

Definition

Leaking of nasal mucus down the throat passage.

Emotional aspect

Swallowed tears and unexpressed feelings.

Reflexes

- As for Nasal Disorders.
- Concentrate on the throat and shoulder reflexes, milking the sides of toes thoroughly to release the 'lump in the throat'.

Other suggestions

- Massage both feet, especially the necks of the toes, with aromatherapy essential oils, to further release from the grips of social constraint: camomile, eucalyptus, fennel, lavender, lemon, rosemary. Also use as an inhalation, as well as in the bath and aromalamps.

Footnote: *Acknowledge and openly express true emotions and feelings.*

ROOT CANAL TREATMENT

See Teeth

SINUSES

Definition

Air cavities within the skull's bony structure that lighten the weight of the head. They are lined with mucous membrane.

Emotional aspect

Space to play around with and mould conscious thoughts.
Sounding boxes for ideas:

Frontal sinuses, between eyebrows, scan the universe for initial inspiration.

Sphenoidal sinuses, immediately below the pituitary gland, intuitively receive thoughts and energise them.

Ethmoidal sinuses, in front of sphenoidal sinuses, bring light and understanding to the realm of thought.

Super-maxillary sinuses of antrums activate and channel thoughts for physical manifestation.

Reflexes

- Sinus reflexes, found on the tips of all toes. Massage to keep the sinuses clear, so that thoughts can be conjured up, taken apart, altered, transformed, played with and related to other images.

Other suggestions

- Smells conjure thoughts and evoke memories.
- Keep a clear head and an open mind for all kinds of possibilities and ideas!

SINUSITIS

Definition

Congestion and inflammation of sinus mucosa, causing extreme discomfort.

Emotional aspect

No space to think because angry, irritable thoughts inflame and irritate the mucosa.

Reflexes

- Central nervous system reflexes, especially the solar plexus reflexes, to open the mind.

- Sinus reflexes for the natural expansion of bone so that congested mucus can be naturally absorbed and expelled.
    Taut skin: congested with irritable thoughts.
    Hard skin: conceals irritability.
    Flaking skin over the hard skin: irritability at having to conceal irritability!
- Eye reflexes for clarity of vision.
- Endocrine system reflexes, especially the pituitary, pineal, thyroid, thymus and adrenal gland reflexes, for emotional calm and tolerance.
- Neck and shoulder reflexes to ease congestion.
- Respiratory reflexes to expand the chest and ease the interchange of energies.
- Liver reflexes for the ability to deal with everything in a more tolerant manner.
- Circulatory, lymphatic and urinary system reflexes to flush through toxic substances and for the free exchange of vibrant life-forces.
- All bodily reflexes (see foot chart) for inner calm and understanding.

Other suggestions

- If severe, seek professional guidance.
- Massage both feet, especially the toe pads, with aromatherapy essential oils, to calm the whole further: eucalyptus, geranium, peppermint, rosemary, thyme. Also use for inhalations and in bath water.
- Natural, wholesome foods avoiding dairy products, alcohol, additives, preservatives, colourants, etc.
- Drink plenty of purified fluids to clear the head and body.
- Relaxation techniques for inner calm and increased tolerance.

STIFF NECK

See Neck Disorders

TEETHING

Definition

Pain, irritability and discomfort as the first teeth erupt.

Emotional aspect

Natural process that gives children the opportunity to make their own decisions.

Reflexes

- See Tooth Disorders.

Other suggestions

- Seek professional guidance if severe.
- Massage both feet with aromatherapy essential oils to soothe inflammation and discomfort further: camomile, lavender, yarrow.
- Give the baby something cool to chew on, e.g. a piece of apple or a teething ring.
- Fresh fruit juice if constipated.
- Raw, unbeaten egg white on the nappy rash, if required.
- Dip cotton wool into an egg cup with one drop of camomile added to a teaspoon of oil and apply directly to the gum.
- Homoeopathic remedies: Aconite – if feverish and acute; Belladonna – for convulsions that arise from teething; Chamomilla – to ease irritability and flushed cheeks; Colocynth – if the child also has colic pains; Nux Vomica – if the child is also constipated.

THROAT DISORDERS

Sore Throats

Tonsillitis

Quinsy

Peritonsillar abscess

Definition

Interference with the natural functioning of the internal tube that eases interaction between the body and the environment.

Sore throat: extreme discomfort, especially when swallowing.
Tonsillitis: acute inflammation of one or both tonsils and surrounding area with festering pus.

Emotional aspect

Social restrictions strangle and stifle expression as well as creativity.

Sore throat: incensed at having to swallow hurtful expressions or from not being able to express true feelings and thoughts.
Tonsillitis: inflamed at having to swallow perceivably unpalatable life experiences.

Reflexes

- Central nervous system reflexes, concentrating on all reflexes, to expand the mind and calm the nerves.
- Throat, neck and shoulder reflexes to release from the grips of fear and to open avenues of expression.
- Endocrine system reflexes, especially the pituitary, pineal, thymus and adrenal gland reflexes, for inner harmony.
- Lymphatic system reflexes, concentrating on the sides and necks of all toes, to soothe the throat reflexes and release emotional congestion.
- Liver reflexes to expel festering emotions.
- Circulatory, lymphatic and urinary system reflexes to eliminate toxic substances for the full expression of life.

Other suggestions

- If severe seek professional guidance.
- Massage both feet, concentrating on the toes pads and necks, with aromatherapy essential oils to accelerate the healing process: bergamot, camomile, cinnamon, eucalyptus, lavender, onion, sandalwood, tea-tree, thyme.
- Swallow life experiences with love and understanding to realise full potential.

- Choose words with care.
- Unconditional love and natural creativity are easily swallowed and expressed!
- Homoeopathic remedies: Aconite – for rough, dry, hoarse, sore throats; Belladonna – to ease red, burning throat, with headache; Hepar. Sulph. – to relieve irritable fish-bone sensation; Mercurius – for hot, dry throat which is making swallowing difficult.
- Raspberry leaf tea gargle to ease symptoms.
- Light, wholesome food to fortify the whole.
- Plenty of purified fluids to flush through life's expressions with ease.
- Bach flower remedies for peace of mind.
- Relaxation techniques for self-confidence.

Footnote: *Those who courageously voice their individual creativity colour the world with their imagination to make a world of difference!*

TINNITUS

Definition

Subjective impression of ringing or roaring sounds in the ears.

Emotional aspect

Subconsciously blocking out other options. Refusing to hear the true self for fear of not being able to cope with the emotional turmoil that may be evoked.

Reflexes

- See Earache.
- Concentrate on the ear reflexes to keep ears open.

Other suggestions

- Seek professional guidance.
- Massage both feet, especially the toe pads and toe necks,

with aromatherapy essential oils for a greater peace of mind:
bergamot, camomile, frankincense, lavender, lemongrass,
peppermint, rosemary.
* Bach flower remedies for self-awareness.

Footnote: *Listen to the inner voice for it can offer peace and
tranquillity.*

TONSILLITIS

See Throat Disorders

TOOTH DISORDERS

Root Canal Treatment

Definition

Erosion of the hard covering of the teeth causes holes and
cavities or obstruction in the root canals depriving the rest of the
tooth of essential life-forces. Extreme discomfort and possible
infection from the exposure of encapsulated nerves and blood
vessels. The acute, dull pain can radiate to the face, eye orbit or
opposite jaw.

Emotional aspect

Extreme uncertainty preventing firm decisions from being made.

Reflexes

* See Mouth Disorders.
* Give extra attention to the teeth, jaw, neck and shoulder
  reflexes to nurture and strengthen the whole.

Other suggestions

* Seek professional guidance.
* Massage both feet, particularly the toe pads, with
  aromatherapy essential oils to further ease discomfort:
  camomile, clove, lemon.

- For toothache, apply to the gum with cotton wool:
    one drop of clove oil or place a clove on the tooth (not
    clove oil for children); or brandy or whisky; or hot
    compress with camomile oil.
- Homoeopathic remedies: Aconite – for relief if aggravated by
  cold; Chamomilla – for severe toothache that is worse at
  night; Merc. Sol – to ease stabbing pains that radiate to the
  ears; Plantago – apply locally or internally for sensitive teeth;
  Silicea – to ease pain aggravated by hot or cold food. Also for
  root abscess or gum boil; Staphysagria – for severe pain.
- Bach flower remedies for self-confidence.

Footnote: *Inner security provides confidence and courage to make
decisions intuitively, founded on universal truth.*

VERTIGO

See Dizziness

WISDOM TEETH

Impacted

Definition

Back molar teeth, which generally appear later in life. Impacted
wisdom teeth, imprisoned in sockets, are not able to break
through the gums.

Emotional aspect

Feeling too insecure for expansive, lateral thoughts.

Reflexes

- As for Mouth Disorders.
- Concentrate on all the toes, especially the big and little toes,
  to expand the mind and ease intense pain.

Other suggestions

- Seek professional guidance.
- Massage both feet, especially the toes, with aromatherapy essential oils to expand the whole further: camomile, calendula, lavender, myrrh.
- Stretch the toes by separating them for expansive thoughts.

Footnote: *Expand thoughts beyond the physical limitations of perception and inspire the world with universal ingenuity and understanding.*

*L*YMPHATIC AND IMMUNE SYSTEMS

LYMPH AND THE LYMPHATIC SYSTEM

Definition

The lymphatic system filters and removes foreign bodies from the body. Lymph vessels travel alongside blood vessels on a more superficial level. Lymph, a transparent fluid, leaves the blood, through the capillary walls, to nurture tissue cells. It then engulfs any foreign or toxic substance within the lymph vessels for eventual elimination from the body via the blood, thereby keeping the body toxin-free.

Emotional aspect

Flushes through old thoughts, feelings and emotions to lighten the load and make way for fresh, progressive concepts.

Reflexes

Lymphatic system reflexes are situated throughout the body and are massaged to purify body contents.

- The milking movement effectively keeps the lymphatic vessels vibrant and clear.

Other suggestions

- Massage both feet with aromatherapy essential oils to further increase the elimination of toxic substances: basil, cypress, fennel, grapefruit, juniper, lemongrass, rosemary.
- Relaxation techniques for the free flow of life-forces.

LYMPHATIC DISORDERS

Definition

Tension interferes with the production, distribution and function of lymph and allows toxins to build up and weigh down the body.

Emotional aspect

Subconsciously feeling bogged down and finding little pleasure and joy in life.

Reflexes

- Central nervous system reflexes to alert the mind and make space for loving, joyful thoughts.
- Endocrine system reflexes, particularly the pituitary, pineal, thymus and adrenal gland reflexes, to reduce vulnerability and for emotional harmony.
- Circulatory system reflexes to encourage the distribution of love and joy throughout.
- Liver reflexes to fire the whole with enthusiasm.
- Lymphatic system reflexes to flush out toxic substances and release hurtful emotions.
- Splenic reflex for the natural production of lymph and inner peace.
- Skeletal system reflexes for the natural develpment of white blood cells.
- All bodily reflexes on both feet for overall immunity and inner strength to cope with anything and everything.

Other suggestions

- See Lymphatic System.
- Seek professional guidance.
- Massage both feet with aromatherapy essential oils: To assist with the elimination of toxic substances: basil, cyprus, fennel, grapefruit, lemongrass, orange. To boost immunity: bergamot, camomile, clary sage geranium, lavender, lemon, sandalwood, vetiver. To accelerate the healing process: camomile, eucalyptus, fennel, geranium, lavender, lemon, rose.
- Plenty of purified fluids, particularly fresh fruit juices, to flush through unwanted wastes.
- Relaxation techniques for in-depth appreciation of the self.
- Do things because you 'want' to, not because you 'have' to. It is amazing how suddenly there are so many things you really *want* to do!

AUTO IMMUNE DISEASE

AIDS

HIV

Definition

The self-destruction of bodily tissue by one's own antibodies, causing muscle wastage and extreme fatigue.

Emotional aspect

Feeling vulnerable, frustrated and inadequate because others appear to condemn and criticise personal values. Inner turmoil, conflict and confusion.

Reflexes

- Physical contact is an essential aspect of the healing process so only avoid open wounds.
- Concentrate on all central nervous system reflexes, especially the brain and solar plexus reflexes, for a total shift in consciousness and self-confidence.
- Spend time on the eye reflexes to see the true self in a more acceptable light.
- Endocrine system reflexes, particularly the pituitary, pineal, thymus and adrenal gland reflexes, for emotional control and the replenishment of natural resources.
- Circulatory and heart reflexes to spread love and joy throughout the whole.
- Liver reflexes to eliminate anger and frustration.
- Muscular reflexes for inner strength.
- Lymphatic and urinary system reflexes for the expulsion of toxic substances and feelings.
- All reflexes on both feet for overall well-being, energy and inner strength.

Other suggestions

- AIDS Society: contact The Terrence Higgins Trust, 52–54 Grays Inn Road, London WC1X 8JU, Telephone: 0171 831 0330, for information and counselling.

- Seek professional guidance.
- Massage both feet and the whole body with aromatherapy essential oils to accelerate the healing process: bergamot, camomile, clary sage, frankincense.
- Wholesome, natural foods to build up bodily strength.
- Detoxification program of raw fruit and vegetables with plenty of purified water to cleanse through the whole.
- Zinc and vitamin C to strengthen immunity.
- Garlic, an anti-viral agent.
- Creative, rewarding activity to boost self-esteem.
- Listen to tapes and read inspirational books on healing the self. *Doors Opening: A Positive Approach to AIDS* video, or *AIDS: A positive Approach/Healing Imagery* audio tape.
- Visualisation, affirmations and meditations to replace perceived threats with unconditional love for the self.
- Fear is the greatest threat and worst enemy. Eliminate it by making a quantum leap in the thought process.
- Bach flower remedies for personal joy and freedom.
- Oxygen or ozone therapy to destroy HIV element.

Footnote: *Aid the self by looking within for true identity so that the soul can find peace, fulfilment and joy on the earth plane.*

CHILDHOOD INFECTIOUS DISEASES

Measles, Chicken-pox, Scarlet Fever, Mumps, etc

Definition

A particular group of diseases with acute fever due to a specific bacteria or virus that run a definite course often in epidemic proportions. They are believed to be highly contagious and generally result in an immunity against further attack. Although more common in childhood, they can occur at any stage in life.

Emotional aspects

Generally perceived to be part of childhood development, but more usually associated with uneasiness due to childish behaviour of adults within the environment.

113

Reflexes

- All central nervous system reflexes, especially the brain and solar plexus reflexes, to ease headaches and pain, to raise the level of consciousness beyond social conditioning and to calm the mind.
- Concentrate on the face, neck and shoulder reflexes to relieve related symptoms such as a dry, furred tongue and sore throat.
- Endocrine system reflexes, particularly the pituitary, pineal, thymus and adrenal gland reflexes to reduce rigors and fevers, and for emotional tranquillity.
- Digestive system to naturalise peristaltic movements so that the appetite is stimulated and constipation is prevented or eased.
- Liver reflexes to release uneasiness and frustration.
- Affected reflexes to release from the grips of anxiety and speed the healing process.
- Circulatory, lymphatic and urinary system reflexes to enhance distribution of essential life-forces and for the natural elimination of toxic substances.
- All bodily reflexes to reduce irritable rashes and skin eruptions and energise the whole.

Other suggestions

- Seek professional guidance.
- Massage both feet, concentrating on the toes and affected reflexes, with aromatherapy essential oils to reduce inflammation further and accelerate healing: camomile, coriander, lavender, lemon, niaouli, tea-tree.
- Also use in inhalations, aromalamps and baths.
- Rest and relaxation techniques to restore the whole.
- See Insomnia for sleeplessness.
- Small quantities of wholesome, nourishing food, as required, to fortify mind, body and soul.
- Plenty of purified fluids for a thorough cleansing.
- Tepid sponge or lukewarm baths to reduce rigors and fevers.
- Mouthwashes with glycothymoline and lemon juice mixed with warm water.

- Homoeopathic remedies: *Chicken-pox* Apis – to relieve itching; Rhus Tox – for the early stage of restlessness; Aconite – to ease the febrile stage of anxiety and fear; Ant. Tart. – to calm vesicle development. *Measles* Euphrasia – to ease streaming nose, eyes and photophobia. Aconite – to reduce high fever, dry cough, restlessness. Pulsatilla – to ease related gastric upsets. *Mumps* Aconite – to reduce fever and restlessness; Pulsatilla – if there is breast or testicle involvement. Belladonna – to ease right-sided parotitis. Rhus Tox – to ease left-sided parotitis.
- Bach flower remedies to restore faith and for reassurance.

Footnote: *Lovingly create space for the self and for others and accept universal protection with joy.*

GLANDULAR FEVER

Mononucleosis

Definition

Infection, of unknown origin, affecting certain white blood cells. Marked lymphatic and glandular involvement causing enlargement and tenderness of the glands, especially in the neck, axillae and groins.

Emotional aspect

Frustration at not feeling appreciated and loved. Lacking in self-worth.

Reflexes

- As for Lymphatic Disorders.
- Concentrate on the endocrine reflexes, particularly the pituitary, pineal, thymus and adrenal gland reflexes, to reduce fevers.
- Lymphatic and glandular reflexes concentrating on the neck, axillae or groin reflexes to reduce swelling and flush through fresh ideas.

Other suggestions

- See Lymphatic Disorders.
- Treat symptoms to ease the discomfort.
- Bed rest to restore the whole.
- Plenty of purified fluids, particularly fresh fruit juices to flush through toxins.
- Homoeopathic remedies: Baryta Carb – to ease general glandular symptoms; Belladonna – to reduce high fever and glandular involvement; Phytolacca – to relieve headaches and glandular swelling.
- Bach flower remedies for self-assurance.

Footnote: *Unconditionally love personal qualities and appreciate personal achievements.*

HODGKIN'S DISEASE

Definition

The progressive malformation of the blood and lymph cells that destroy harmful micro-organisms in the body, with the gradual enlargement of glands.

Emotional aspect

Subconscious belief of being personally inadequate and not able to meet expectations.

Reflexes

- As for Lymphatic Disorders.
- Circulatory system reflexes to encourage the distribution of love and joy throughout the whole.
- Lymphatic and urinary system reflexes.

Other suggestions

- See Lymphatic Disorders.
- Inform the local health visitor and social worker.
- Partake in a pleasurable pursuit that gives joy and a sense of achievement.

INFECTION

Definition

The invasion of the body by an organism that causes inflammatory changes or disease.

Emotional aspect

A built-up reaction to annoying, irritating or frustrating factors that are angrily manifested physically within the body.

Reflexes

- Concentrate on all central nervous system reflexes for a calm, clear, open mind to release pain and fever.
- Endocrine system reflexes, particularly the pituitary, pineal, thymus and adrenal gland reflexes, for emotional control.
- Liver reflexes to release accumulated toxic emotions.
- All bodily reflexes on both feet, with particular attention to afflicted areas (see foot chart) to calm the body's overall reaction to infuriating factors.

Other suggestions

- See Lymphatic Disorders.
- Spring-clean the house, office, school desk, etc. for the physical release of outdated articles.
- Plenty of purified water and fresh fruit juices to flush out the whole.
- Homoeopathic remedies: Aconite – reduce infection, redness, swelling and fever. Hypericum tincture – apply locally during early onset; Silicea – to ease chronic pus infection; Staphysagria – to ease excruciating pain with itching, anger and resentment.

LUPUS

Definition

An auto-immune condition in which antibodies attack their own tissue.

Emotional aspect

Subconscious emotional self-destruction due to poor self-worth and self-esteem.

Reflexes

- As for Lymphatic Disorders.
- Spend time on central nervous system, especially the brain and solar plexus reflexes, to reduce depression, lethargy and fatigue by improving the perception of the self and expanding the mind inwardly and outwardly so that a balance can be achieved.
- Lymphatic system reflexes, concentrating on the node reflexes, to prevent killer T-cells from destroying their own bodily tissue.
- Muscular and skeletal system reflexes increase mobility and muscular strength.
- Circulatory and urinary reflexes for the free flow of essential life-forces to counteract any weight loss or anaemia and eliminate all toxic substances.

Other suggestions

- Lupus U.K., 51 North Street, Romford, Essex RM1 1BA. Tel: 0708 731251.
- See Lymphatic Disorders.
- Protect the skin if sensitive to the sun.
- Exercises to strengthen the whole.

Footnote: *Life is a valuable possession to be treasured and cared for.*

NODES AND NODULES

Definition

Small swellings and protuberances, with smaller nodules.

Emotional aspect

The accumulation of extreme frustration, built-up resentment and compounded hurts. Generally work-related.

Reflexes

- As for Lymphatic Disorders.
- Concentrate on circulatory, lymphatic and urinary system reflexes for an ongoing cycle of energy and enthusiasm.
- Specific reflexes of the affected area (see foot chart) to allow space for swellings to be absorbed and eliminated from the whole.

Other suggestions

- See Lymphatic Disorders.

Footnote: *Success is perception meeting opportunity with joy and enthusiasm.*

VIRAL INFECTION

See also Infection

Definition

A minute living organism, a virus, that causes diseases such as influenza, measles and polio-myelitis.

Emotional aspect

Resentment at the hardships of life.

Reflexes

- See Infection.

Other suggestions

- See Infection and Lymphatic Disorders.
- Massage both feet with aromatherapy oils containing anti-viral properties: cinnamon, clove, eucalyptus, garlic, lavender, onion, oregano, ravensara, sandalwood, tea-tree, thyme.
- Supplements and vitamins to boost immunity.

Footnote: *Hardships provide an opportunity for self-development.*

CIRCULATORY SYSTEM

CIRCULATION

Definition

The circular course of blood and lymph to nourish bodily cells with essential life-forces and to remove toxic substances to keep mind, body and soul in peak condition.

Emotional aspect

Circulation is enhanced and blood vessels expand with feelings of love and joy. Tension, unhappiness and destructive emotions squeeze the blood vessels and constrict the natural flow of life depriving them of this vibrancy and energy.

Reflexes

- Blood vessel reflexes are found throughout both feet. Massage for the free distribution of essential life-forces for enthusiasm and vitality.

Blood circulation

(1) Head reflexes and toes:	Circulate loving, joyful thoughts.
(2) Neck reflexes and big toes:	Circulate the expression of love and joy.
(3) Chest reflexes on the balls of both feet and the second toes:	Circulate feelings of love and joy.
(4) Upper digestive reflexes on the upper half of the instep and the third toes:	Actively circulate love and joy.
(5) Lower digestive reflexes on the lower half of the instep and the fourth toes:	Circulate the exchange of love and joy through communication and health.
(6) The pelvic reflexes on the balls of the feet and the fifth toes:	Circulate the security of love and joy.

Other suggestions

- Massage both feet with aromatherapy essential oils to stimulate circulation further: basil, bergamot, black pepper, cardamom, clary sage, geranium, ginger, hyssop, rose, rosemary.
- Herbal remedies to ease the flow: ginger root tea; lime flower herbal tea; nettle herb tea or broth.
- Homoeopathic remedies: Carbo Veg. – the best remedy for cold, blue extremities. Lachesis – to improve purple extremities. Pulsatilla – for heat intolerance.
- Exercise to strengthen the whole.
- Relaxation techniques to ease circulation.
- Bach flower remedies for confidence and reassurance.

Footnote: *Circulate freely to experience the exciting, ever-changing adventure of life with love and joy.*

BLOOD AND CIRCULATORY DISORDERS

Definition

Interference with the free blood flow, or with the composition of blood corpuscles or in the utilisation of blood.

Emotional aspects

Subconsciously inhibiting the flow and distribution of unconditional love and joy throughout the body due to fear, anxiety, disappointment or distrust.

Reflexes

- Concentrate on all central nervous system reflexes, to increase drive and initiative.
- Endocrine system reflexes, stimulating each reflex well, to reactivate the emotional need for self-preservation.
- Circulatory reflexes, especially the heart reflexes, to ease the flow of life throughout the whole.
- Respiratory system to increase oxygen intake and reduce any breathlessness.

- Arm and leg reflexes to improve circulation and reduce the incidence of 'pins and needles'.
- Skeletal reflexes to encourage the natural production and formation of blood corpuscles.
- Liver reflexes to release accumulated emotions.
- Lymphatic and urinary system reflexes to eliminate toxic and inhibiting substances.
- All bodily reflexes on both feet for inner strength and vitality.

Characteristic reflexes

- Taut, red feet: feeling under pressure, which long term can interfere with the blood circulation and blood development.
- White, flaccid feet: drained of energy due to tension.
- Swollen feet: weighed down by the enormity of life clogging the channels of love and joy.

Other suggestions

- Homoeopathic remedies: Carbo Veg. – for ice-cold, blue extremities; Lachesis – to relieve purple extremities; Pulsatilla – for heat intolerance.

Footnote: *Happiness comes from within, so don't wait for others to make you happy, create it for yourself!*

ANAEMIA

Definition

Poor quality or an insufficient number of red blood cells and haemoglobin due to: an inadequate production, poor development, lack of distribution, incomplete utilisation, the over destruction of the blood cells, or an excessive loss through bleeding. Pallor, weakness, tiredness, breathlessness, lack of drive and initiative arise from the inadequate distribution of oxygen throughout the body.

Emotional aspects

Apathy towards life in general.

Reflexes

- As for Blood and Circulatory Disorders.
- Circulatory and heart reflexes for release from the grips of anxiety for the free flow of blood to enhance the distribution of oxygen.
- Respiratory system reflexes to increase oxygen intake and reduce breathlessness.

Other suggestions

- See Circulatory Disorders.
- Seek professional guidance, especially if pregnant.
- Wholesome, natural foods, rich in iron, such as dark-leaved vegetables, dried fruit, wholemeal bread as well as those filled with vitamin B and folic acid, such as milk, eggs, cheese, carrots, avocado pears, pumpkins, melons, torula yeast.
- Vitamin and mineral supplements, particularly vitamin B12, folic acid and iron, to further fortify the whole.
- Herbal remedies: Agrimony, lady's Mantle, nettle tea, Swedish Bitters.
- Homoeopathic remedies: Ferrum Met. – restores the natural glow; Arsenicum – to boost bodily resources; Phosphorus – to enhance self-confidence.

Footnote: *Unconditional love and joy bolster confidence and enthusiasm for life.*

ANGINA

Definition

A tight strangling sensation, severe cramping or extreme pain that grips the chest and radiates down the left arm. Tension restricts the blood flow to the heart muscle depriving it of oxygen and essential life-forces.

Emotional aspect

Highly strung. Worriers. Overly concerned about other's feelings and what they may think.

Reflexes

- See Myocardial Infarction.

Other suggestions

- See Myocardial Infarction and Circulatory Disorders.
- Stop and rest during an attack.
- Avoid strenuous exertion.
- If overweight find why you are having to overprotect yourself emotionally so that weight can be reduced to relieve any strain on the heart.
- Bach flower remedies, especially Rescue Remedy, during an attack, to ease the discomfort and for the strength to cope.

Footnote: *No one is a threat unless allowed to be!*

ARTERIOSCLEROSIS

See also Cholesterol

Definition

The gradual loss of arterial elasticity due to deposits thickening blood vessel walls. The increased pressure required to force blood through the restricted lumen causes hypertension (high blood pressure) and deprives the cells of essential life-forces, vitality and vibrancy.

Emotional aspect

Strictness with self. Lack of elasticity or inflexibility of thought.

Reflexes

- As for Blood and Circulatory Disorders.
- Spend time on the liver, circulatory and lymphatic reflexes to release from the shackles of self-constraint and to clear the blood vessels.

Other suggestions

- See Circulatory and Blood Disorders.
- Relaxation and deep-breathing techniques to open the mind and the heart.
- Enjoyable, non-competitive exercise for renewed energy and vitality.
- Creative, rewarding activity that gives pleasure.

Footnote: *Those who give with unconditional love and joy, receive abundant love and joy!*

BLOOD CLOTTING

Definition

Coagulation of blood within the vessels due to tension constricting the blood vessels and slowing down the blood flow as vast volumes of blood try to squeeze along narrowed lumens.

Emotional aspect

Gripping tension from unresolved emotional conflict blocking the way.

Reflexes

- As for Blood and Circulatory Disorders.

Caution: A large clot, once released from the grips of tension, can travel to the brain causing a stroke, or to the heart causing a heart attack. *To my knowledge this has not happened,* but the recipient **must** be made aware of the possibility and given a choice.

- Concentrate on the circulatory system, concentrating on the heart reflexes, to release from the grips of terror and to make way for a healthy, strong blood flow.

125

Other suggestions

- See Blood and Circulatory Disorders.
- Herbal remedies: Aloe, grape, mustard, wild strawberries.

Footnote: *Liberate the soul from the bondage of the mind!*

CARPAL–TUNNEL SYNDROME

Definition

Extreme tension in the carpus, the bony connection between the hand and forearm. The blood flow is drastically constricted due to tension depriving the hand nerves and muscles of essential life-forces causing intermittent or constant excruciating pain.

Emotional aspect

Subconsciously feeling insecure. Frustrated at not keeping a grip on things.

Reflexes

- As for Blood and Circulatory Disorders.
- Spend time on the arm and hand reflexes to release from the grips of tension, anxiety and frustration.

Other suggestions

- Massage both feet, concentrating on the affected reflexes, with aromatherapy essential oils to ease tension further: eucalyptus, lavender, marjoram. Also massage both hands, the arms and shoulders at least twice a day.

Footnote: *The justice and balance of cosmic law is within everyone's reach.*

BLOOD VESSELS
HEART

See also Circulation

Definition

The circular course of blood through a massive network of large and small tubes. Under natural pressure from a hollow muscular organ, the heart, a continuous flow of blood is distributed to nourish and fortify all bodily cells, as well as remove toxic substances for elimination from the body, thereby maintaining a balance.

Emotional aspect

Distribution of love and joy throughout to cherish and support life for inner harmony. The warm, kind and gentle hearted have plenty of love for themselves and others.

Reflexes

Blood vessel reflexes are situated throughout the feet. See foot chart for exact reflex of specific vessels. Massage to enhance the exchange of natural life-forces and the natural distribution of unconditional love and joy throughout.

Characteristic circulatory reflexes

- Skin colour indicates blood flow and related emotions, both of which are subject to constant change. Emotion has an immediate effect on the blood flow as indicated by the variety of colouring on the feet revealing varied and possibly conflicting emotions throughout the whole.

  Flesh colour: a healthy, vibrant blood flow and happy, relaxed emotions.
  White: drained of energy and enthusiasm slowing down blood distribution and the process of life.
  Red: angry or embarrassed bringing blood vessels to the surface.
  Blue: feeling cold from emotions having been inhibited, battered or hurt restricting the presence of love and joy.
  Yellow: from feeling fed-up with a jaundiced view of life, leaving little enthusiasm or energy.
  Green: restricted blood flow due to envy.

The **Heart reflexes** are minute swellings, which are sometimes well embedded under the skin's surface, immediately below hard balls on insides of both feet. Massage to expand and strengthen loving emotions.

Characteristic heart reflexes

Vibrant and healthy: full of love and joy.
Swollen: filled with heartache.
Flat and white: drained of emotion.
Red: angry and frustrated regarding matters of the heart.
Broken blood vessels: bleeding, broken heart.

Other suggestions

- Enjoy wholesome, natural foods to fortify the whole.
- Drink plenty of purified fluids for ongoing circulation.
- Relaxation techniques to establish contact with true self.
- Herbal remedies for healthy circulation: Ginger root tea; Lime flower tea; Nettle herb tea.

Footnote: *Life is an ongoing cycle of unconditional love that keeps the world going around!*

CHOLESTEROL

Definition

Non-saponifiable fat, found within nervous tissue, red blood corpuscles, animal fat and bile which, during times of stress, clogs blood vessels.

Emotional aspect

Resistance to the natural flow of love and joy due to past emotional trauma or fear of experiencing disappointment again.

Reflexes

- As for Blood and Circulatory Disorders.
- Spend time on the circulatory, lymphatic and urinary system

reflexes to release toxic substances and for the uninhibited distribution of love and joy.

- All bodily reflexes for the natural utilisation of nutritional substances.

Other suggestions

- See Blood and Circulatory Disorders.
- Enjoy wholesome, natural foods eliminating fats to energise the whole.
- Oxygen or ozone therapy to ease areas of congestion.

Footnote: *Receive and give unconditional love and joy.*

CORONARY THROMBOSIS

See Heart Attack

COMMON COLD

See Upper Respiratory Tract Infection

HEART DISORDERS

Heart Attack

Cardiac Arrest

Myocardial Infarction

Coronary Thrombosis

Definition

Little or no heart functioning due to poor or inadequate supply of essential life-forces to the cardiac tissue, especially the muscles.

Emotional aspect

The heart is the centre of love and is very susceptible to changing moods. Feelings of emotional deprivation squeeze love, joy and vitality from the heart, whilst fear and anxiety grip it tightly, robbing it of its mobility. Severe emotional trauma can break the heart.

Reflexes

- Central nervous system reflexes, especially the big, second and third toes, as well as the midbrain (for cardiac centre) and solar plexus reflexes to release body from the grips of fear and anxiety.
- Endocrine system, concentrating on all reflexes, for emotional control, inner peace and harmony.
- Neck and shoulder reflexes to take the weight off the shoulders.
- Circulatory and heart reflexes to strengthen and make space for expansion.
- Respiratory system reflexes to relieve dyspnoea, cyanosis and congested feeling within lung, for natural expansion and contraction.
- Digestive system reflexes to ease stomach and intestinal congestion and naturalise digestive processes.
- All bodily reflexes for overall well-being.

Other suggestions

- Seek professional guidance immediately.
- Inform the local authorities, the health visitor and the social worker.
- Bed rest initially.
- Tune into body's needs and meet them accordingly.
- Partake in pleasurable pursuits that give joy and sense of achievement.
- Enjoy a regular intake of small quantities of wholesome, natural foods as required to fortify the whole.
- Relaxation techniques for inner tranquillity.
- As strength increases, introduce passive exercises.

- Bach flower remedies, especially Rescue Remedy, for inner strength and understanding.
- See Circulation.

Footnote: Fill the heart with loving feelings for the self and for others.

HODGKIN'S DISEASE

See page 116 in the section on The Lymphatic and Immune Systems.

Footnote: Life is a gift, enjoy it!

HYPERGLYCAEMIA

See Diabetes

HYPERTENSION

See also Blood and Circulatory Diseases

Definition
Raised blood pressure causing headaches, giddiness, tinnitus or epistaxis (nose bleeds) due to tension.

Essential hypertension: no complications.
Malignant hypertension: starts at an early age and can be very severe.
Portal hypertension: due to tension in the portal blood system, generally due to hepatic cirrhosis.

Emotional aspect
Persistent mental pressure. Hypersensitivity. Many unresolved issues that have created internal pressure.

Reflexes
- As for Blood and Circulatory Disorders.

- Spend time on the eye, nose, neck and shoulder reflexes to encourage a free exchange of energies.
- Digestive system reflexes, specifically the liver and stomach reflexes, for ability to cope.

Other suggestions

- See Blood and Circulatory Disorders.
- Avoid excessive alcohol which interferes with the natural flow of blood.
- Stop smoking to remove the smokescreen and acknowledge true emotions.

HYPOGLYCAEMIA

Definition

A lack of sugar/glucose in the blood. If diabetic, an attack is preceded by sweating, palpitations, mental confusion, trembling, hunger and weakness.

Emotional aspect

Feeling overwhelmed and drained by the enormity of life and a feeling that it lacks sweetness.

Reflexes

- See Blood and Circulatory Disorders.
- Concentrate on liver reflexes to release disappointments and frustrations.

Other suggestions

- See Blood and Circulatory Disorders.
- Tune into the body's nutritional requirement and eat regular small quantities of wholesome natural foods for a continual release of energy.

Footnote: *Active involvement in meeting all obligations with a sincere desire, rather than being compelled to, generates ongoing energy and an enthusiasm for life.*

LEUKAEMIA

Definition

The excessive production or immature formation of white blood corpuscles from a swollen spleen, enlarged lymphatic glands or diseased bone marrow. Short- or long-term affliction with lengthy periods of remission.

Emotional aspect

Subconscious hopelessness. Destruction of creativity.

Reflexes

- Central nervous system reflexes, concentrating on all reflexes, to boost morale and release the mind from self-imposed limitations.
- Endocrine system reflexes, stimulating each reflex well, to reactivate the emotional need for self-preservation.
- Liver reflexes to release accumulated destructive feelings.
- Lymphatic system reflexes for the natural production of white blood cells and to flush out excessive white blood cells as well as other toxic substances.
- Splenic reflex to reduce the tendency towards obsessive behaviour.
- Circulatory reflexes, especially over the long bone reflexes, to encourage the natural formation of blood in the bone marrow, as well as to ease the flow of life throughout the whole.
- All bodily reflexes on both feet for inner strength and vitality.

Other suggestions

- See Blood and Circulatory Disorders.
- Tune into the body's needs and meet them accordingly.
- Pleasurable pursuits that give joy and sense of achievement.

Footnote: *Expand the thought process, to acknowledge all talents fully, with gratitude and joy.*

MYOCARDIAL INFARCTION

Heart Attack

Definition

The death of part of the heart muscle due to tension, which diminishes the blood supply and deprives the area concerned of its essential nutrients.

Emotional aspect

Subconscious perception of deprivation of love and understanding from long-standing emotional conflict. Fear and anxiety clutch it tightly, restrict its mobility, and deprive it of essential life-forces.

Reflexes

- As for Blood and Circulatory Disorders.
- Spend time on the circulatory and heart reflexes to free from the grips of fear, anxiety or greed and to ease expansion and functioning of the whole.
- Lymphatic system reflexes to let go of dependency and obsession with material assets and relax the whole musculature.

Other suggestions

- Bed rest initially.
- Tune into the body's needs and meet them accordingly.
- Enjoy pleasurable pursuits that give joy and a sense of achievement.
- Regular intake of small quantities of wholesome, natural foods as required to nourish the whole.

Footnote: *Unconditionally love the self and others so that full meaning and expression can be given to life.*

PALPITATIONS

Definition

Awareness of the heart pounding in the chest often with a

sense of panic and anxiety. Can be experienced during pregnancy.

Emotional aspect

Hypersensitivity and overcome with emotion.

Reflexes

- As for Blood and Circulatory Disorders.
- Concentrate on the respiratory reflexes, particularly the diaphragmatic reflexes, to calm the anxiety.
- Heart reflexes for the natural expansion and contraction of the heart.

Other suggestions

- See Blood and Circulatory Disorders.
- Homoeopathic remedies: Nux vomica – if there is also indigestion, constipation and irritability; Spigelia – the treatment of choice.

Footnote: *Faith in the universal order of life is intuitively reassuring.*

PHLEBITIS

Definition

Inflammation of the venous channels with possible blood clotting, known as thrombosis.

Emotional aspect

Anger and frustration at being denied the opportunity to enjoy life to the full.

Reflexes

- As for Blood and Circulatory Disorders.
- Concentrate on the liver reflexes to release anger and frustration.
- Leg reflexes to reduce oedema, pain, tenderness and the incapacity for increased mobility.

Other suggestions

- See Blood and Circulatory Disorders.
- Rest with the legs elevated.
- Homoeopathic remedies: Arnica – either locally or internally if associated with trauma; Belladonna – to ease inflammation; Hamamelis – either locally or internally if associated with varicose veins; Pulsatilla – to relieve discomfort and heat intolerance.

Footnote: Create inner happiness and joy by looking within for the fountain of truth, self-love and acceptance!

SICKLE CELL ANAEMIA

Definition

A blood disorder. The naturally rounded, pliable red blood cells are rigid and half-moon shaped and have a limited capacity to carry oxygen, which deprives bodily cells of their essential life-forces. Common in malaria-infected countries.

Emotional aspect

Conforming to restrictive belief systems denies the whole of love and joy.

Reflexes

- Central nervous system, especially the big, second and third toes, to calm the nerves, ease the pain and expand the mind to embrace loving, joyful perceptions.
- Concentrate on the eye reflexes to prevent future complications, as well as enhance vision and intuition.
- Endocrine system reflexes, concentrating on the pituitary, pineal, thymus and adrenal gland reflexes, for emotional security and inner peace.
- Digestive system reflexes, specifically the liver and stomach reflexes, for the natural secretion of the intrinsic factor for the full utilisation of vitamin B12 for the maturation of red blood cells.

- Muscular reflexes, particularly the neck and shoulder, as well as the circulatory system reflexes to ease the grip of anxiety on the musculature for the free blood flow to nurture the whole.
- Bone reflexes, especially the sternum, skull and the end of the long bone reflexes for ideal environment for healthy red blood cell formation.
- Lymphatic and urinary system reflexes for the elimination of toxic substances particularly malformed red blood cells, at the end of the 120 day cycle, so that they can be replaced with vibrant, healthy new cells.

Other suggestions

- Sickle Cell Society, 54 Station Road, Harlesden, London NW10 4UA. Tel: 0181-802 0994
- Sickle Cell Anaemia Relief, 148A Chiswick High Road, London W4 1PR. Tel: 0181-954 8045/7990
- Wholesome natural nutrients, with milk, egg and cheese for vitamin B12 and folic acid intake to encourage healthy cell formation and functioning.
- Vitamin B complex for increased vitality.
- See Blood and Circulatory Disorders.

Footnote: *Fully expand to embrace all of life's possibilities with love and joy.*

THALASSAEMIA

Definition

A lack of haemoglobin in the blood causing severe anaemia. Monthly blood transfusions are required to build up iron in the liver or, in severe cases, a bone marrow transplant may be required. More common in Mediterranean climates.

Emotional aspect

An inhibited capacity to accept life with unconditional love and joy.

Reflexes

- See Sickle Cell Anaemia.

Other suggestions

- Thalassaemia Society, 107 Nightingale Lane, Hornsey, London N8 7QY. Tel: 0181-348 0437
- See Blood and Circulatory Disorders.

Footnote: *Live life to the full!*

VARICOSE VEINS

Definition

Swollen, dilated veins, usually in the legs, but also in the anal region (known as haemorrhoids). Occasionally experienced during pregnancy.

Emotional aspect

Feeling pressurised and weighed down by responsibilities and burdens. Unhappy about certain aspects of the present situation.

Reflexes

- As for Blood and Circulatory Disorders.
- Spend time on the liver reflexes to unburden concern for self and others.
- Leg reflexes to ease from the grips of torturous anxiety and to promote healing.
- Circulatory reflexes for the free exchange of love and joy throughout the whole.

Other suggestions

- See Blood and Circulatory Disorders.
- Foot baths with geranium and lavender.
- Relaxation techniques to ease pressure.
- Use support stockings or tights.
- Wholesome, natural food, especially if overweight.

- Homoeopathic remedies: Ac. Fluor – for simple, uncomplicated varicose veins; Hamamelis Tinc. – local application when acute; Pulsatilla – after childbirth; Silicea – if complications with inflammation.

Footnote: *Life is a pleasure – enjoy doing things for the fun of it!*

*r*ESPIRATORY SYSTEM

Definition

The passages and organs that assist with the interchange of gases between the atmosphere and the body to substantiate life. The rhythmic expansion and contraction of the respiratory muscles allows for stability and a harmonious relationship between the internal and external environments.

Emotional aspect

Harmonious interaction between the self and atmospheric conditions. Ability to adapt to environmental conditions depends on feelings of self-worth and self-esteem. Breast and chest reflexes overlap because the type of nurturing influences feelings about the self.

Reflexes

Nose reflexes, on the outer joints of big toes, are massaged to filter and warm the atmospheric air to ease the exchange of gases, as well as for self-recognition. They vibrate to turquoise/purple.

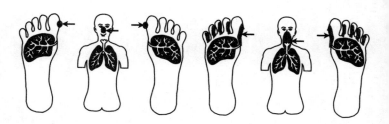

Nose reflexes

Trachea & Laryngeal reflexes

Trachea and Laryngeal reflexes, stretch from the nose reflexes along the outer edge of both feet to halfway along the hard balls and are massaged to facilitate the movement of air in and out of the body. They vibrate to blue/turquoise.

Bronchial and Bronchiole reflexes, branch all over the hard balls of both feet and are massaged for the even distribution of environmental air and for the natural release of internal gases. They vibrate to green.

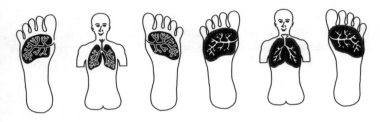

Bronchi & Bronchiole reflexes   *Lung reflexes*

Lung reflexes, on the hard balls of both feet, are massaged for the full expansion and exchange of gases, by relaxing the surrounding musculature. They vibrate to green.

Diaphragmatic reflexes, on the division between the hard balls and the insteps, are massaged for the ability to adapt and to soothe the emotions of the solar plexus. They vibrate to green/yellow.

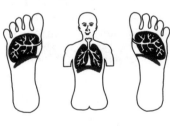

Diaphragm reflexes

Characteristic reflexes

Swollen balls: filled with unresolved emotion.
Hard balls: putting up a resistance rather than giving into feelings.
Shiny balls: friction of emotions and feelings within the environment.
Hard skin over balls: to protect self-identity and own space.

141

Other suggestions

- Massage both feet with aromatherapy essential oils for the full expansion of breath: eucalyptus, geranium, lavender, lemon, peppermint.
- Periodically take in full breaths, hold them, and then slowly release them.
- Aromatic warm baths, with deep breathing, to expand the airways.
- Yoga breathing exercises for the full utilisation of the breath.
- Rebirthing and relaxation techniques for the subconscious release of suppressed emotions.
- If atmospheric air had to be paid for, more attention would be paid to breathing!

Footnote: *Allow the breath of life to expand beyond physical limitations to incorporate the whole.*

BREATHING AND RESPIRATORY DISORDERS

Definition

Inflammation, stricture and spasm interfere with the natural absorption and utilisation of fresh atmospheric air or the release of toxic substances in the form of carbon dioxide.

Emotional aspect

Disturbing emotions and intense concentration temporarily halt breathing, particularly in life-threatening situations. Disease occurs when long-term distress, fear or anxiety, continually interfere with the rhythmic pattern of expansion and contraction. Irritating emotional factors throw it into spasm.

Reflexes

- Central nervous system reflexes, particularly the big and second toes, as well as the midbrain and solar plexus reflexes, to expand the mind and calm nerves.
- Endocrine system reflexes, especially the pituitary, pineal, thyroid and thymus gland reflexes, for emotional equilibrium.

- Neck and shoulder reflexes to relax the upper musculature.
- Respiratory system, concentrating on the diaphragmatic reflexes, for general homoeostasis.
- Breast reflexes for self-confidence and ease of interaction within the environment.
- Heart reflexes to expand the heart with unconditional love for the self and others.
- Circulatory, lymphatic and urinary system reflexes for the natural distribution of essential life-forces and the elimination of toxic wastes.
- Digestive tract to stimulate the appetite and nourish the whole.
- Arm reflexes for increased mobility and accommodation of the whole.

Other suggestions

- Seek professional guidance.
- Aromatic essential oil inhalations, to open and clear nasal and airway passages, to assist in the relief of rhinitis (inflamed nasal passages with runny nose and sneezing), sputum or phlegm: camomile, cinnamon, eucalyptus, frankincense, ginger, hyssop, lavender, nutmeg, red thyme, rosemary, tea-tree. To relax the musculature: frankincense, geranium, jasmin, rose. Also use to massage the feet, especially the toes and hard balls.
- Sneezing eliminates minor irritations, whilst coughs and haemoptysis (coughing up blood) release deep-seated, hidden emotions. These symptoms should never be suppressed, but eased through reflexology, relaxation and the use of inhalations.
- Relaxation techniques to expand the chest.
- Light, wholesome nutrients to fortify the whole.
- Vitamin and mineral supplements.
- Plenty of purified fluids.
- Bed rest.
- Sleep with head propped up on several pillows.
- Regular deep breathing, especially for pain, dyspnoea or cyanosis (bluish colour).

- Wear loose clothing to ease the expansion and contraction of chest.
- Prop up in bed to facilitate breathing.
- Create a well-ventilated, warm environment.
- Thyme tea for chest infections.
- Bach flower remedies to release fear of everyday life.

Footnote: *Fill the whole with confidence, love and joy for life.*

ASPHYXIA

Definition

Choking and suffocation due to the lack of breath which temporarily interrupts respiration.

Emotional aspect

Panic and extreme fear of inadequacy. Feeling claustrophobic.

Reflexes

- As for Breathing and Respiratory Disorders.
- **During an attack** immediately place both thumbs on the solar plexus reflexes for as long as required. It may take one minute to half an hour to ease an attack!

Other suggestions

- See Breathing and Respiratory Disorders.
- During an attack, concentrate on taking in deep rhythmic breaths to relax all bodily muscles, particularly the ribcage.
- Deep, expansive breaths periodically throughout the day.
- Escape to open places, such as the country, whenever possible.
- Bach flower remedies especially Rescue Remedy **during an attack** for immediate reassurance, inner strength and encouragement.

Footnote: *Open up to life's possibilities and embrace them with enthusiasm.*

ASTHMA

STATUS ASTHMATICUS

Definition

Overly sensitive bronchial tubes that narrow and go into spasm, hampering expiration. Possible inflammation.

Cardiac asthma: mainly at night and associated with left-sided heart failure and pulmonary congestion.
Renal asthma: accompanies kidney disease.

Emotional aspect

Triggered off by emotional upset or hypersensitivity. Fear of not being able to breathe for the self.

Cardiac asthma: mistrust of love and life's processes.
Renal asthma: follows severe disappointment that takes the breath away.

Reflexes

- As for Breathing and Respiratory Disorders.
- **During an attack** (Status asthmaticus) Immediately place both thumbs on the solar plexus reflexes.
- Concentrate on the respiratory tract reflexes, concentrating on the airway diaphragmatic reflexes, to relax spasm of the smooth muscle and to reduce the swelling of the mucosal lining and create space for regular, expansive breathing.

Other suggestions

- See Breathing and Respiratory Disorders.
- National Asthma Campaign, Providence House, Providence Place, London N1 0NT.
- Bach flower remedies, especially Rescue Remedy **during an attack** for immediate reassurance and inner strength.
- Herbal remedies: garlic, honeysuckle, mint, pawpaw, mistletoe.
- Homoeopathic remedies: Phosphorus – to reassure and expand bronchi; Kali Carb. – to ease early morning and evening wheezing; Medorrhinum – to relieve difficult recurrent attacks only. Arsenicum – to ease anxiety.

BRONCHITIS

Definition

Acute or chronic infection and inflammation of the mucosal lining of the bronchi.

Acute bronchitis: sudden attack of short duration.
Chronic bronchitis: ongoing attacks of acute bronchitis.

Emotional aspect

Anger or frustration within the environment. The conflict can also simmer beneath the surface to erupt at a later stage.

Reflexes

- As for Breathing and Respiratory Disorders.
- Concentrate on the respiratory system, concentrating on the bronchial and diaphragmatic reflexes, to expand the tubes and ease the exchange of gases.
- Neck, breast and shoulder reflexes to facilitate interaction within the environment.

Other suggestions

- See Breathing and Respiratory Disorders.
- Seek professional guidance.
- Homoeopathic remedies: Aconite – for the first 24-hours to ease short, dry cough, irritation and raised temperature; Bryonia – to ease a violent, dry, painful cough with headaches and chest pains; Belladonna – if accompanied by high temperature that is worse at night; Ant. Tart – to eliminate loose, rattling moist mucus.

UPPER RESPIRATORY TRACT INFECTION

COLDS

Acute Coryza

Definition

Inflamed irritability of the upper airway mucosa. Streams of mucus pour from the nasal cavity, accompanied by general malaise.

Emotional

Confused and feeling out of control with so many commitments all at once.

Reflexes

- As for Breathing and Respiratory Disorders.
- Concentrate on facial reflexes, especially the nose reflexes, to reduce irritability and ease mucosa secretions.
- Neck and throat reflexes to release from the grips of tension.

Other suggestions

- Massage both feet, especially the toes and hard balls, with aromatherapy oils to ease tightness and relieve congestion further: eucalyptus, lavender, tea-tree. Also use in bath and inhalations.
- Place a small bowl of boiling water with three drops of eucalyptus by the bed, particularly at night, to ease congestion.
- Cleanse the whole with fresh fruit and pure fruit juices for at least one day.
- Drink plenty of purified fluids.
- Camomile herb tea with sage, lime flower herbal tea, rosemary tea.
- Rest.
- Bach flower remedies to ease congestion.

Footnote: *Make a fresh start – flush out the old to create space for new, more creative ideas!*

COUGHS

Definition

The violent, noisy expulsion of air from the lungs, with or without mucus. Spasmodic contractions of the diaphragm triggered off by an infection or foreign body irritating the respiratory tract.

Emotional aspect

Subconscious release of swallowed, congested emotion. Extreme nervousness.

Reflexes

- As for Breathing and Respiratory Disorders.
- Concentrate on the respiratory reflexes, concentrating on the airway reflexes, to release from the grips of tension and to allow the free flow of mucus, to clear the airway.
- Liver reflexes for the subconscious release of congested emotions.

Other suggestions

- See Breathing and Respiratory Disorders.
- Drink plenty of purified water to flush through congestion.
- Homoeopathic remedies: Aconite – to ease a constant dry cough that is worse at night; Belladonna – to relieve violent attacks of shaking coughing; Bryonia – to ease a dry cough that is worse during the day; Hepar Sulph – to improve coughs that are due to an infection; Sulphur – to ease moist rattling coughs.
- Vitamin and mineral supplements to build up strength and resistance.

CROUP

Definition

Spasmodic dyspnoea with a harsh cough and stridor, associated with spasm or inflammation of the larynx. Usually affects young children.

Emotional aspect

Subconscious fear and inability to take in the enormity of life.

Reflexes

- As for Breathing and Respiratory Disorders.

- Massage the feet of both parents and the child. It is important for the parents to stay calm at all times so as not to alarm the child.
- Spend time on the neck and shoulder reflexes to make space.
- Respiratory reflexes, concentrating on the air passages and diaphragmatic reflexes, to release from the grips of tension and to allow the free exchange of life-forces.

Other suggestions

- See Breathing and Respiratory Disorders.
- Seek immediate professional guidance.
- Boil a kettle in the room for steam to keep the airways moist and expanded. Remember to keep topping up the water!
- Keep calm!
- Bach flower remedies, especially Rescue Remedy for all concerned, for the ability to cope.
- Relaxation techniques particularly for the parents.

EMPHYSEMA

Definition

Change in the elasticity of tissue causing distension and thinning of tissues, particularly in the lungs. Unnatural presence of air in bodily tissues or cavities, either due to the introduction of air or gas through perforation or incision, or when the alveoli lose their elasticity due to disease.

Emotional aspect

Hopelessness at the enormity of life's expectations.
Overwhelming feeling of little or no self-worth.

Reflexes

- As for Breathing and Respiratory Disorders.
- Spend time on respiratory reflexes, concentrating on the diaphragm reflexes, to relax chest muscles for ease of movement.

Other suggestions

- See Breathing and Respiratory Disorders.

HYPERVENTILATION

Definition

Rapid breathing lowering amount of dissolved carbon dioxide in the blood plasma, causing alkalinity and 'pins and needles'.

Emotional aspect

Panic and frustration with present situation. Resisting the natural flow of life and reluctant to change due to a deep fear and insecurity. Overcome by emotions.

Reflexes

- As for Breathing and Respiratory Disorders.
- Concentrate on the respiratory system reflexes, particularly the neck, shoulders and diaphragmatic reflexes, to release the chest from the grips of terror.
- Liver reflexes for the subconscious release of extreme panic.

Other suggestions

- See Breathing and Respiratory Disorders.
- Cup hands around the nose and mouth to breathe in exhaled air and to prevent carbon dioxide deprivation. The correct proportions of carbon dioxide assist the natural functioning of the respiratory centre.

LUNG DISORDERS

Definition

Interference with a section of the respiratory process, inhibiting or preventing the complete exchange of gases, depriving the body of oxygen and allowing carbon dioxide to build up.

Emotional aspect

Intense concentration and disturbing emotions temporarily halt breathing, particularly in perceived life-threatening circumstances. Distress, anxiety, grief, fear and feelings of inadequacy disturb the rhythmic expansion and contraction of lungs. Short-term the body copes but long-term it causes disease.

Reflexes

- As for Breathing and Respiratory Disorders.
- Spend time on the respiratory tract reflexes, concentrating on the lung, shoulder and diaphragm reflexes, for the rhythmic movement of lungs.

Other suggestions

- See Breathing and Respiratory System.

PNEUMONIA

Definition

Inflammation of one or both lungs due to various micro-organisms.

    Broncho-pneumonia: scattered inflammation.

    Lobar pneumonia: only one lobe affected.

    Tuberculous pneumonia: uncommon these days.

    Viral pneumonia: caused by a virus rather than bacteria.

Emotional aspect

Suppressed anger at the threat to feelings of self-worth and self-esteem. No more energy to deal with life's demands.

Reflexes

- As for Breathing and Respiratory Disorders.
- Concentrate on the respiratory system reflexes, specifically the lung reflexes, to release from the grips of desperation and to allow for natural expansion.
- Liver reflexes to release suppressed anger.

Other suggestions

- See Breathing and Respiratory Disorders.
- Create a well-ventilated, warm environment.

Footnote: *Life is a possession to be valued, so hang on to it!*

$\mathcal{D}$IGESTIVE SYSTEM

Definition

The organs and passages involved with the break down, assimilation and absorption of food, to provide nutritional substances for energy and new cell formation.

Emotional aspect

The emotional ability to bite off life's experiences, bit by bit, chew on them and break them down into acceptable, manageable sized proportions for the absorption to energise the whole for inner growth and development.

Reflexes

Regular reflexology massage attunes mind, body and soul to specific nutritional needs so that ultimately food is consumed only to replace natural energy and replenish cells as required. This eliminates the excessive intake of food and enables surplus weight to be released.

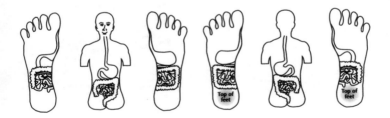

Digestive reflexes (Primary - soles)   Digestive reflexes (Secondary - tops)

The Mouth reflexes, found below the outer joints of both big toes, as well as on all the little toes, are massaged to naturalise mobility so that contents can be expansively accommodated. They vibrate to turquoise/purple.

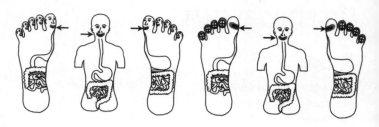

Mouth reflexes   *Teeth reflexes*

The Teeth reflexes, found on the toe pads below the outer joints of both big toes, as well as on all the little toes, are massaged to strengthen and ease decision making. They vibrate to turquoise/purple.

The Tongue reflexes, found on the toe pads below the outer joints of both big toes, as well as on the little toes, are massaged for mobility, strength and sensitivity. They vibrate to turquoise/purple.

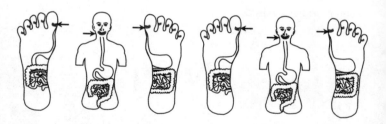

Tongue reflexes   *Salivary glands*

The Salivary Gland reflexes, found on the toe pads below the outer joints of both big toes, as well as on the little toes, are massaged to facilitate the breakdown of food particles. They vibrate to turquoise/purple.

The Throat reflexes extend from the outer joints of both big toes along the inner edge of both feet to the lower crease below the big toe and are massaged for flexibility, ease of expansion and to enhance the two way exchange of energies. They vibrate to turquoise/blue.

The Oesophagus reflexes extend from the outer joints of both big toes along the inner aspects of both feet to the bases of the hard balls and are massaged for relaxed, effective peristalsis. They vibrate to turquoise/green.

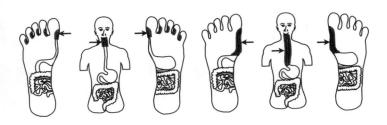

Throat reflexes   *Oesophageal reflexes*

The Cardiac Sphincter reflexes, situated at the bases of the hard balls of the feet, are massaged to relax this muscular opening at entrance of the stomach. They vibrate to green.

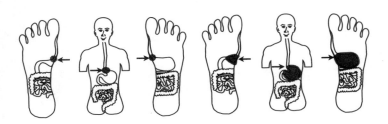

Cardiac sphincter reflexes   *Stomach reflexes*

The Stomach reflexes are found mostly on the inner half of the upper **left** instep with a smaller portion on the inner half of the upper **right** instep. They are massaged to harmonise the kneading activity and the natural outpouring of gastric acid so that food and personal experiences can be easily broken down for inner growth and development. They vibrate to yellow.

The Pyloric Sphincter reflex, found only on the **right** foot, midway between the centre and inner edge, immediately below the hard ball of the foot, is massaged to relax the muscular ring at the exit of the stomach to ease the expulsion of stomach contents. It vibrates to yellow.

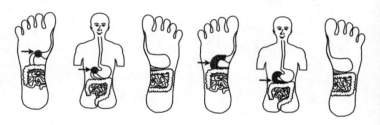

Pyloric sphincter reflexes   *Duodenal reflexes*

The Duodenum reflex is 'C' shaped and is found in the upper inner quarter of the **right** instep only. It is massaged to naturalise peristalsis and create a receptive environment for pancreatic and gall bladder secretions and for the active breakdown of food and life's experiences. It vibrates to yellow/orange.

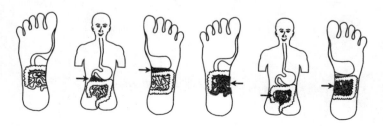

Ileum reflexes   *Small intestine glands*

The Ileum reflex is a short strip from the inner edge to the centre of the **left** foot, immediately above the waistline and is massaged to ease the passage of the contents from the stomach to the intestines. It vibrates to yellow/orange.

The Small Intestinal reflexes, occupy the lower half of the instep on both feet and are massaged to encourage the natural absorption of nutrients into the bloodstream to nurture the whole. They vibrate to yellow/orange

The Ileo-caecal Valve reflex, situated in the lower left corner of the fleshy **right** instep is massaged to ease the flow of waste products through this muscular sphincter from the small intestine to the large colon. It vibrates to orange/red.

The Appendix Vermiformis reflex situated in the lower, outer corner of the **right** instep is massaged so that it stays healthy, by separating good from bad, and remains out of harm's way. It vibrates to orange/red.

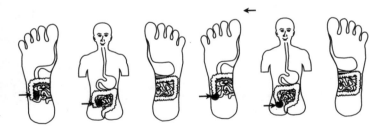

Ileo-caecal valve reflexes   *Appendix reflexes*

The Ascending Colon reflex is situated along the outer edge of the **right** fleshy instep as far as the waistline, and vibrates to yellow/orange.

The Hepatic Flexure reflex is a palpable swelling halfway along the outer edge of the **right** fleshy instep and vibrates to yellow/orange.

157

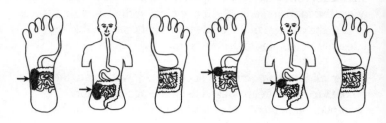

Ascending colon reflexes *Hepatic flexure reflexes*

The Transverse Colon reflexes situated across the waistline of both feet, climb slightly towards the end of reflexes on the **left foot**. They vibrate to yellow/orange.

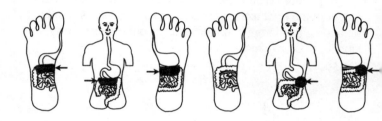

Transverse colon reflexes *Splenic flexure reflexes*

The Splenic Flexure reflex, which is just above the waistline on the outer edge of the **left** fleshy instep, vibrates to yellow/orange.

The Descending Colon reflex along the outer edge of the **left** fleshy instep, from waistline to heel, vibrates to yellow/orange.

The Sigmoid Colon reflex along the lower edge of the **left** fleshy instep, vibrates to orange/red.

The Rectum reflexes, on the arc on the inner edges of both feet, extend from the end of the sigmoid colon reflex to the hollows, midway between the tips of the heels and the inner ankles. They vibrate to orange/red.

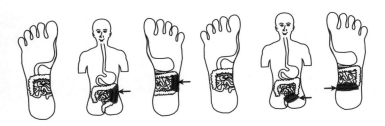

Descending colon reflexes   Sigmoid colon glands

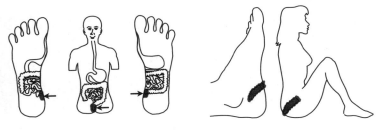

Rectum reflexes

Rectum reflexes

The Anal reflexes, midway between the inner ankle-bones and the tips of the heels, vibrate to red.

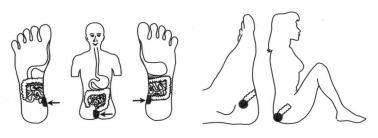

Anal reflexes

Anal reflexes

All the reflexes from the **Ileo-Caecal Valve** to the **Anal reflexes** are massaged for the free movement and easy expulsion of bodily wastes in their natural form of faeces. This provides the whole with the welcome relief of absorbing that which is necessary and letting go of that which would otherwise be burdensome.

The Liver reflexes, found mainly on **right** foot, is a triangular area occupying the upper outer **right** instep with a small wedge on the upper inner **left** instep, immediately below hard ball of the foot. It is massaged for the natural ability to continually assimilate, metabolise, break down, build up, store and eliminate many different substances all at the same time, especially at night-time. They vibrate to yellow/orange.

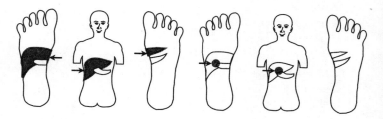

Liver reflexes   *Gall-bladder reflexes*

The Gall-bladder reflex is a tiny ball-like palpable swelling just above the waistline and slightly off centre, towards the outer edge of the **right** foot. It is massaged for the effective storage and release of bile and bitter emotions that no longer have value. It vibrates to yellow/orange.

The Pancreas reflexes, situated immediately above the waistlines on the inner halves of both feet, are massaged for the smooth flow and sweetness of life. They vibrate to yellow.

Pancreas reflexes

Other suggestions

Food, like experiences, energises the body and gives it the strength to deal admirably with any situation that comes its way.

- Eat what **your** body requires, when **your** body requires it, in quantities **your** body needs.
- Natural, wholesome foods contain natural energy and no artificial substances.
- Keep a balance! Eat primarily to satisfy bodily needs, but also to occasionally pamper the taste buds!
- Accept food with peace of mind and sincere appreciation.
- Ideally eat in solitude or in happy, relaxed surroundings.
- Energise food before eating by holding your hands over the food directing life-forces and energy into its fibre.
- Chew food well.
- Fennel, centaury or peppermint teas aid and improve digestion.
- Life is an exciting journey with testing points along the way. These enhance personal growth and development. Take in all opportunities and then decide what is palatable and beneficial and eliminate the rest.

DIGESTIVE DISORDERS

Definition

Interruption of or interference with the natural process of accepting food into the body for nourishment and energy, depriving the whole of its life force.

Emotional aspect

Intense emotions interfere with the natural ability to bite off life's experiences, to stomach situations, absorb all that is going on and release that which is not required.

Reflexes

Massage all digestive reflexes to naturalise digestive abilities to take in and deal with life's experiences with ease.

- Central nervous system reflexes, particularly the big, third and fourth toes, as well as the solar plexus reflexes, to release subconscious pressure and calm the mind.
- Endocrine system reflexes for emotional peace and reassurance.
- Digestive system reflexes, especially the liver and colon reflexes, for inner harmony.
- Liver reflexes to release feelings of inadequacy and frustration for inner hermony.
- Circulatory, lymphatic and urinary reflexes to flush through toxic substances.
- All reflexes on both feet for inner strength and to energise the whole.

Unnatural reflexes

Temporary congestion arises from perceived obstacles in life's present circumstances

- Hard skin over the **mouth** reflexes from having to keep the mouth shut with the possibility of overcompensating with food.
- A hard ridge of skin down the **oesophageal** reflexes indicates difficulty in having to continually swallow unpalatable situations.
- Swollen **cardiac sphincter** reflexes indicate a possible hiatus hernia or heartburn.
- Flat, lifeless **stomach** reflexes indicate exhaustion or having to give in because there is too much to stomach.
- Swollen **stomach** reflexes arise from feeling bloated or indicate difficulty in stomaching all that is going on.
- A swollen **pyloric sphincter** reflex indicates an inability to progress with ease due to some past emotion holding back efforts.
- Swollen **duodenal** reflexes indicate a resistance to the flow of life.
- Sunken, pale **small intestinal** reflexes indicate exhaustion from having to absorb so much.
- The **small intestine** reflexes swell when there is a feeling of being overwhelmed with so much going on.

- Flattened **colon** reflexes arise from a feeling of being defeated.
- **Colon** reflexes swell from trying to please so many people by being better than the best.
- Drained **rectum** and **anal** reflexes suggest a perceived need to escape an unpleasant situation.
- **Rectum** and **anus** reflexes swell when they are clogged up from hanging on to outdated belief systems and ideas.
- Taut **liver** reflexes indicate exhaustion from repeatedly giving vent to aggressive emotions and feelings.
- Puffy, red **liver** reflexes are storing anger, frustration and disappointment.
- If the **gall-bladder** reflex is too sensitive to touch, allow the third finger to hover over the reflex for as long as can be tolerated to allow bitterness to dissipate.
- **Pancreatic** reflexes swell when there is a craving for sugar to replace the sweetness that is perceived to be lacking from life.
- Flattened **pancreatic** reflexes imply a feeling of being drained of life's sweetness.

Other suggestions

- See Digestive System.
- Seek professional guidance.
- Regular cleansing with fresh fruit juices for one to three days to flush through toxic substances.
- Aromatherapy essential oils. To enhance well-being: camomile, geranium, jasmine, lavender, rose, rosemary; to flush through toxic substances: clary-sage, fennel, geranium, jasmine, lavender, lemongrass; for inner calm: camomile, eucalyptus, fennel, frankincense, geranium, hyssop, lavender, lemon, peppermint, rose, rosemary; to naturalise peristalsis: lemon, peppermint, rosemary; to revitalise the whole: cypress, eucalyptus, geranium, ginger, hyssop, lavender; to ease discomfort: coriander, cypress, grapefruit.
- Enjoy regular, small meals of wholesome, natural foods to nurture the whole.
- Consider vitamin and mineral supplements to boost vitality.

- Drink plenty of purified liquids daily.
- Relaxation techniques for inner calm.
- Bach flower remedies for total harmony.

ABDOMINAL CRAMPS AND COLIC

Definition

The involuntary, slow, forceful contraction of the abdominal muscles with severe constriction and spasm of the smooth muscle of the intestinal wall.

Emotional aspect

Anxiety and undue pressure from high expectations of self.

Reflexes

- As for Digestive Disorders.
- Digestive system reflexes, especially the liver and colon reflexes, for inner harmony.

Other suggestions

- See Digestive Disorders.
- Breathe into the contractions.

ANAL DISORDERS

Definition

Extreme tension, severe laxity or inflammation interfere with the natural expansion and contraction of the anal muscle.

Anal abscess: a pocket of pus in the anus.

Anorectal bleeding: bleeding from the rectum via the anus, or from haemorrhoids.

Anal fissure: a painful crack in the mucous membrane generally due to hard faeces.

Pruritis ani: anal irritation and uncomfortable sensitivity of the anal channel.

Emotional aspect

Insecurity and a reluctance to release the past, leading to anger and frustration at being weighed down by the load.

Anal abscess: built-up anger at not being able to let go of past emotions.

Anorectal bleeding: frustration and sadness at feeling overburdened and weighed down by past traumatic emotions.

Anal fissure: hardened faeces carry hurtful, useless emotions that create friction and prevent complete evacuation.

Anal irritation: discomfort of past actions.

Reflexes

- As for Digestive Disorders.
- Spend time on the digestive tract reflexes, concentrating on the liver and anal reflexes to relax muscular tension and to ease elimination of outdated emotions.

Other suggestions

- See Digestive Disorders.
- It is easier to let go of things that have no value. Outdated emotions hamper progress, so release them with love and understanding.
- Eat natural foods especially those with a high roughage content.
- Drink plenty of natural fluids.
- Abdominal muscle exercises to massage the colon and assist with the passage of faeces.
- Bach flower remedies for peace of mind.
- Herbal supplements: Black Forest tea; Licorice.
- Cough when defecating, to relax the anal muscles and facilitate faecal progress.

ANOREXIA AND ANOREXIA NERVOSA

Definition

Anorexia: loss of appetite.

Anorexia nervosa: a nervous disorder and a symptom of hysteria that causes extreme emaciation and a confused body image.

Emotional aspect

Anorexia: a temporary disinterest in eating.
Anorexia nervosa: eating away at the self. Total rejection of
life due to deep fear or a profound dislike of the self.

Reflexes

- As for Digestive Disorders.
- Concentrate on the central nervous system reflexes,
  especially the big, second and third toes, as well as the solar
  plexus reflexes, to alter the perception of the self and life.
- Digestive tract reflexes, especially the liver reflexes, for inner
  tranquillity.
- Lymphatic and urinary system reflexes to eliminate deep fear
  and distrust.

Other suggestions

- See Digestive Disorders.
- Give unconditional love, support and understanding to the
  self and others.
- Enjoy appetising, wholesome, nourishing foods in small
  quantities at frequent intervals to encourage a gradual build-
  up of confidence.
- Add grapefruit, orange or lemon aromatherapy essential oils
  to the food.
- Homoeopathic remedies: Argent Nit. – to improve self-
  esteem; Natrum Mur. – for general well-being; Silicea – for
  cold, sweaty extremities.

Footnote: *Every life has meaning – find that meaning and live life
to the full.*

APPENDICITIS

Definition

Acute pain, inflammation and tenderness of the appendix
vermiformis and its surrounding areas. If allowed to build up it
can ultimately burst.

Emotional aspect

Profound anger and resistance to life's good aspects due to ingrained fear.

Reflexes

- As for Digestive Disorders.
- Concentrate on the digestive tract reflexes, particularly the appendix and liver reflexes, to release from the grips of terror.

Other suggestions

- See Digestive Disorders.
- Relax abdominal muscles and breathe deeply.
- Homoeopathic remedies for grumbling appendix: Apis – to relieve stinging, burning pain; Bryonia – to ease movement; Lachesis – for relief from the cutting pain that is worse on waking.

Footnote: Unconditional love of life and absolute faith in the Truth leaves no space for anger.

BOWEL DISORDERS

Definition

Tension or laxity interfere with the natural peristalsis and movement of intestinal contents.

Emotional aspects

Congestion, from a reluctance or difficulty in releasing built-up emotions, blocks the tubes and weighs down the soul.

Reflexes

- As for Digestive Disorders.
- Concentrate on the central nervous system reflexes, particularly the big, fourth and little toes, as well as the solar plexus reflexes, to motivate natural subconscious decisions as to what to absorb and what to release.

- Digestive system reflexes, especially the bowel and liver reflexes, for inner calm.

Other suggestions

- See Anal Disorders.
- Enjoy wholesome natural foods.
- Drink plenty of purified fluids.

BULIMIA

Definition

Voracious hunger and eating followed by self-induced vomiting.

Emotional aspect

The attempt to force into oneself all of life's experiences and then to purge the body due to self-contempt.

Reflexes

- See Digestive Disorders.
- Digestive system reflexes, concentrating on stomach reflexes, to reduce sensitivity and promote healing.
- Liver reflexes to release self-contempt.

Other suggestions

- See Anorexia.

Footnote: *Take one step at a time to savour the beauty of life and the self.*

CHOLECYSTITIS

GALLSTONES

Definition

Acute or chronic inflammation with calculus formation in the form of stones in the gall-bladder. Severe spasms of colic pain.

Emotional aspect

Angry, embittered thoughts of vexation and humiliation.

Reflexes

- Central nervous system reflexes, concentrating on all reflexes, to ease excruciating pain and release embittered thoughts.
- Endocrine system reflexes, spending time on all reflexes, for emotional equilibrium.
- All digestive tract reflexes, especially: the cardiac sphincter reflexes, to ease heartburn; the oesophageal reflexes, to relieve nausea and flatulence; the stomach reflexes, for dyspepsia; the duodenal reflexes, to ease the release of bile; the bowel reflexes, for lower flatulence.
- Liver and gall-bladder reflexes and urinary reflexes to ease the release of gallstones.
- All bodily reflexes for overall well-being.

Other suggestions

- See Digestive Disorders.
- Tune into the body's needs and meet them accordingly.
- Plenty of purified fluids to flush through the system.
- Homoeopathic remedies: Berberis Tinc. – every 5 to 10 minutes to relax spasm; Chelidonium – for all gallstone disorders; Mag. Carb – to ease gripping pain; Veratrum Album – to relieve excruciating pain with cold sweats and considerable flatulence.

CONSTIPATION

Definition

Incomplete or infrequent action of the bowel either due to poor muscle tone or spasm.

Emotional aspects

Faeces, as waste products, represent outdated (wasted) ideas which should be released regularly. Physical, emotional or spiritual insecurity leads to a perceived need to hang on to old beliefs or material possessions.

Reflexes

- As for Digestive Disorders.
- Spend time on the digestive system reflexes, concentrating on the colon, rectal and anal reflexes, for the natural expansion of muscles to ease the expulsion of faeces.
- Liver reflexes for the active release of wasted substances.

Other suggestions

- See Digestive Disorders.
- Avoid laxatives and artificial remedies so that natural bowel movements can be re-instated.
- Homoeopathic remedies: Bryonia – to facilitate passage of faeces; Nux Vomica – for a long-standing situation.
- Include a high fibre intake to provide bulk for faecal movement.
- Drink plenty of purified water to flush through waste matter.
- Black Forest tea to clear digestive tract.

Footnote: *Progress and self-actualisation can only occur with change – new clothes, new car, new ideas, new attitudes!*

DIABETES

Definition

Imbalanced carbohydrate metabolism.

Diabetes insipidus: extreme thirst, increased urine, weight loss and exhaustion.
Diabetes mellitus: insufficient insulin from pancreas, with sugar in the urine.
Hyperglycaemia: too much sugar in the blood.
Hypoglycaemia: blood sugar falls too low.
Diabetic coma: loss of consciousness due to imbalanced blood sugar content.

Emotional aspect

Diabetes occurs 18 months to two years after an emotionally traumatic experience which is perceived to have drained life of its vitality and sweetness.

Reflexes

For best results, massage both feet one hour prior to the administration of insulin or any other drug. Blood or urine sugar content should be tested before and after the treatment to appreciate the incredible effect of reflexology in balancing blood sugars.

- Central nervous system, especially the big and third toes, as well as solar plexus reflexes, to calm the mind.
- Concentrate on the eye reflexes for a clearer view of life.
- Endocrine system reflexes, particularly the pituitary, pineal, thyroid, thymus and adrenal gland reflexes for emotional control and inner understanding.
- Digestive reflexes to improve carbohydrate metabolism, reduce great thirst and counteract extreme hunger and weight loss.
- Pancreatic reflexes to release from the grips of sadness so that functions can naturalise.
- Urinary system reflexes, specifically the kidney reflexes, to control urine and sugar output.
- Circulatory and lymphatic system reflexes to eliminate toxic wastes, improve blood flow and make space for the enhanced distribution of essential life-forces.

Other suggestions

- See Digestive Disorders.
- Regular, wholesome, natural foods.
- Drink plenty of purified fluids.
- Carry glucose sweets or tablets to counteract hypoglycaemia.

Footnote: *Yesterday is past and the future depends on enjoying and appreciating the here and now today.*

DIARRHOEA

Definition

Excessive and frequent discharge of loose unformed faecal matter. Often offensive and sometimes with slime and blood.

Emotional aspect

Fearful, sometimes gripping, anxiety or not able to accept particular circumstances. Running away from the self.

Reflexes

- As for Digestive Disorders.
- Spend time on the digestive reflexes, concentrating on the liver, colon, rectum and anal reflexes, to calm spasms of anxiety and naturalise functions.

Other suggestions

- See Digestive Disorders.
- Drink plenty of purified fluids as well as raspberry leaf tea.
- Enjoy a regular wholesome, appetising food intake.
- Homoeopathic remedies: Arsenicum – for severe diarrhoea with burning, watery stools and mucus; China – for pale, mucusy faeces with possible discharge; Pulsatilla – if also feeling weepy.

Footnote: *Fears are creations of the mind and can be replaced with loving thoughts!*

DYSENTERY

Definition

Acute inflammation of the colon, with ulceration in severe cases, and the frequent passage of mucus and blood-stained stools.

Emotional aspect

Anxiety and frustration at being overwhelmed and hindered by others.

Reflexes

- As for Digestive Disorders.
- Spend time on the digestive system, concentrating on the liver and colon reflexes, to reduce inflammation.
- Build up immunity and replenish the whole with essential nutrients.

Other suggestions

- See Digestive Disorders.

DYSPEPSIA

See Indigestion

FAT

OBESITY

Definition

Fat is a natural component of the body. Excessive fat deposits throughout create added weight to the body, providing surplus covering and protection.

Emotional aspect

A need to protect the self due to extreme sensitivity, fear, insecurity, uncertainty, self-doubt, vulnerability, lack of fulfilment or deep hurt.

Fat arms: frustration at not being able to express the self expansively particularly in the matters of love.
Expansive abdomen: protection against being punched in the stomach or frustrated at not being nourished or able to nurture new life.
Large hips: to prevent security from being threatened.
Fat thighs: the build up of childhood frustrations.
Swollen ankles: prohibiting the pleasures of life.

Reflexes

- As for Digestive Disorders.
- Reflexology effectively controls obesity by releasing the fear and anxieties that the body is subconsciously protecting itself against. The mind becomes acutely aware of its true requirements, thereby reducing dependency on food for comfort.
- Spend time on the central nervous system reflexes, concentrating on all reflexes, to ease fear, anxiety, frustration, insecurity and to build up self-confidence.
- Liver reflexes to release the excessive internal build-up of emotion, frustration and fear.
- Circulatory, lymphatic and urinary system reflexes to eliminate surplus substances and replace with vibrancy.

Other suggestions

- See Digestive Disorders.
- Massage both feet and the body with aromatherapy essential body oils to help relax the musculature so that excessive fats can be absorbed and eliminated from the whole: basil, fennel, grapefruit, juniper, lavender, lemongrass.
- We are **what** we eat and **how** we eat it!
- Eat with joy in the heart and a smile on the face!
- Decide whether food is being eaten to nurture and refuel the body or to satisfy taste buds.
- Use a side plate instead of a dinner plate.
- Chew food well.
- When hungry between meals, enjoy raw fruit and vegetables.
- Eat wholesome, natural foods for vibrant energy.
- Drink plenty of purified fluids to flush through excess substances.
- Spring-clean the home, office, workshed, etc., throwing out old, unused items. Releasing outdated, old physical belongings eases the elimination of tired, unnecessary emotions.
- Homoeopathic remedies: Natrum Mur – to ease the retention of urine; Phytolacca berry – to reduce the craving for food substantially.

- Bach flower remedies for the ability to cope.

Footnote: *Protection comes from within. Nourish the self with unconditional love and joy. No one or nothing is a threat unless allowed to be.*

FLATULENCE
GASTRIC FLATULENCE

Definition
Presence of excessive gas in the digestive tract and a sensation of being bloated and distorted after meals.

Emotional aspect
Extreme fear regarding communication or relationships tenses the body and creates build-up of emotion.

Reflexes
- As for Digestive Disorders.
- Concentrate on the digestive tract reflexes, especially the stomach, colon and liver reflexes, to relax the whole system for natural digestion.

Other suggestions
- See Digestive Disorders.
- Peppermint tea.
- Eat slowly with love and gratitude.
- Homoeopathic remedies: Argent nit. – to ease abdominal pain with flatulence; Carbo veg. – for upper abdominal discomfort; Lycopodium – for lower abdominal discomfort.

FOOD POISONING

Definition
Unnatural reaction to a food substance.

Emotional aspect

Feeling defenceless and vulnerable.

Reflexes

- As for Digestive Disorders.
- Concentrate on the digestive system reflexes, especially the stomach and liver reflexes, to release internal tension and allow food and circumstances to be digested naturally.
- Lymphatic system reflexes to drain away toxic substances.
- All reflexes on both feet for inner strength and to energise the whole.

Other suggestions

- See Digestive Disorders.
- Drink plenty of purified fluids to counteract dehydration.
- Sip castor oil dissolved in warm water, mixed with lemon juice and a drop of peppermint.
- Homoeopathic remedies: Arsenicum – for extreme chill and weakness; Bryonia – to relieve nausea, vomiting, colic and diarrhoea; Carbo veg. – to ease nausea, vomiting, constipated stool, cramping, flatulence and distended bowel; Nux vomica – to calm irritability.
- Determine which experiences are subconsciously repulsive and deal with the situation accordingly.

GASTRITIS

Definition

Inflammation of the mucous membrane lining of the stomach.
　　Acute: due to abuse or bacterial.
　　Chronic: from prolonged dietary indiscretions.

Emotional aspect

Anger and frustration at not being able to 'stomach' certain aspects of life. Emotions affect type, quantity and method of food consumed. This directly affects physical aspects which outwardly express subconscious feelings.

Reflexes

- As for Digestive Disorders.
- Spend time on the digestive tract, particularly the stomach reflexes, to harmonise natural expansion and contraction to promote digestion.
- Liver reflexes to release inflamed emotions.

Other suggestions

- Seek professional guidance immediately.
- Massage both feet, especially the toes and insteps, with aromatherapy essential oils for increased inner calm: camomile, eucalyptus, geranium, lavender, lemon, peppermint, rose, rosemary, tea-tree, thyme.
- See Digestive Disorders.

GAS PAINS

See Flatulence

HAEMORRHOIDS

Definition

Dilated rectal/anal blood vessels that may bleed on defecation due to proximity to the skin's surface. Aggravated by constipation and pregnancy.

Emotional aspect

Feeling pressurised. Anxiety and frustration at having security threatened by overburdening pressures.

Reflexes

- As for Digestive Disorders.
- Spend time on the digestive tract reflexes, concentrating on the rectal/anal reflexes, to release tension and allow the blood vessels to relax back to their natural position.
- Liver reflexes for the release of congested emotions.

Other suggestions

- See Digestive Disorders.
- Homoeopathic remedies: Aloe – for protruding haemorrhoids; Collinsonia – the most useful remedy, especially for marked itching; Nux vomica – for associated indigestion, irritability and constipation; Pulsatilla – useful during pregnancy; Sulphur – if constipated and itchy, but no bleeding.

Footnote: *Time is elastic in the present, creating space for all that is desirable.*

HEARTBURN

Pyrosis

Definition

Burning sensation rising from the stomach to the throat. Tension prevents complete closure of the cardiac sphincter, allowing gastric acid to escape from the stomach into the oesophagus.

Emotional aspect

Extreme anxiety and gripping fear at the possibility of not coping or meeting expectations.

Reflexes

- As for Digestive Disorders.
- Concentrate on the digestive tract reflexes, especially the stomach and cardiac sphincter reflexes, for relaxation and harmony.

Other suggestions

- See Digestive Disorders.
- Have a regular intake of small quantities of wholesome, natural foods as required, avoiding large meals before bed.
- Relaxation techniques.
- Exercise on an empty stomach.

- Bend both knees to pick up objects from a lower level.
- Sleep in a propped up position on several pillows.

HEPATITIS

Definition

Various types of liver inflammation due to a viral infection, toxic drugs or poisons.

Emotional aspect

A resistance to change and suppressed emotions of anger, fear and hatred.

Reflexes

- As for Digestive Disorders.
- Concentrate on the eye reflexes, especially if they are yellow, for a clearer view of life and liver reflexes to release stored emotions and for inner calm.

Other suggestions

- See Digestive Disorders.
- Stay in bed for complete rest.
- Take in small quantities of light wholesome, natural foods as required.
- Drink plenty of purified fluids, with glucose, if the appetite is poor.
- Avoid alcohol, caffeine, nicotine, drugs and fats.
- Use calamine for severe itching of the skin.

ILEITIS

Crohn's disease

Definition

An inflamed ileum with acute pain.

Emotional aspect

Possible dissatisfaction with the self for failing to meet high expectations.

Reflexes

- As for Digestive Disorders.
- Concentrate on the ileo-caecal valve and bowel reflexes, to calm irritable peristaltic movements.

Other suggestions

- See Digestive Disorders.
- Consume frequent, small, wholesome meals initially.
- Use cornflour and soya-bean flour instead of wheat flour during the acute stages.
- Vitamin A, D, B complex, K and calcium supplements to fortify the whole.
- Avoid alcohol, caffeine, nicotine, drugs and fats.

Footnote: *Individuality is the greatest gift to mankind, so overcome self-imposed limitations and accept your own self-worth.*

INDIGESTION

DYSPEPSIA

Definition

Pain, discomfort and difficulty in digesting food.

Emotional aspect

Fear, anxiety, worry, distress and dread prevent adequate digestion or the ability to cope with life's events.

Reflexes

- As for Digestive Disorders.
- Central nervous system reflexes, especially the solar plexus reflexes, to calm the nerves and for clarity of the mind.
- Endocrine system reflex, concentrating on all reflexes, for inner peace.

- Concentrate on the stomach reflexes, to pacify movement to ease digestion.
- All bodily reflexes on both feet for the free distribution and absorption of digested contents and ideas.

Other suggestions

- See Digestive Disorders.
- Take in small, regular amounts of nutritious digestible foods.
- Eat slowly and chew thoroughly.
- Check dentures are well-fitting.
- Consider vitamin and mineral supplements to boost vitality.
- Peppermint and rosemary herbal tea.
- Avoid alcohol, caffeine, nicotine, drugs and fats.
- Relaxation techniques to reduce worry and anxiety.
- Bach flower remedies, especially Rescue Remedy, to ease the mind.
- Homoeopathic remedies: Arsenicum – for weakness, exhaustion and lack of appetite; Calc. carb. – to relieve constant distaste; Natrum Mur – to ease nervous strain and tension, heartburn and upper abdominal pain; Sulphur – for chronic dyspepsia and offensive taste.

INTESTINAL DISEASES

Definition

Diseases of the lower part of the alimentary canal from the pyloric sphincter at the exit of the stomach to the anus.

Emotional aspect

Difficulty in breaking down, absorbing and letting go of certain aspects of life.

Reflexes

- See Digestive Disorders..
- Concentrate on the intestinal tract reflexes, to relax the muscles for the natural assimilation, absorption and elimination of intestinal contents.
- Liver reflexes for the release of inhibiting emotions.

Other suggestions

- See Indigestion.

Footnote: *Go with the flow! Intuitively body, mind and soul know how to assimilate, what to absorb and how much to release.*

JAUNDICE

Definition

Yellow discoloration of the skin and conjunctivae.
Obstructive jaundice: an obstructed gall-bladder with bile-pigment in the blood.
Haemolytic jaundice: the excessive destruction of red blood cells.

Emotional aspect

A jaundiced view on life due to unreasonable prejudices, anger, envy or jealousy.

Reflexes

- As for Digestive Disorders.
- Concentrate on the eye reflexes for a clearer view of life and on the liver, gall-bladder and spleen reflexes, to release aggressive emotions for harmonious functions.

Other suggestions

- See Cholecystitis and Gallstones.

MOUTH DISORDERS

Definition

Interference with the functions of mastication or vocal utterances.
Stomatitis: inflammation of mucous membrane.
Glossitis: inflammation of the tongue.
Mouth ulcers: minor viral infection.

Emotional aspect

Inability to express the self openly and honestly. Reluctance to accept new ideas due to rigidity of thought from fearful insecurity.

Stomatitis: anger at having to keep the mouth shut!
Glossitis: frustration at not being able to roll about ideas with the tongue.
Mouth ulcers: eating away at the self.

Reflexes

- Concentrate on the facial reflexes, especially the mouth and tongue reflexes for free expression.

Other suggestions

- Oral hygiene to keep the mouth fresh and free of encumbrances.
- Mouthwash with one or more aromatherapy essential oils mixed with warm water: geranium, lemon, peppermint and thyme.
- Apply directly to the ulcer: camomile and thyme.

MUCOUS COLON

Definition

Excessive amounts of mucus clog the colon, resulting in impacted faeces and constipation.

Emotional aspect

Stuck in the past and buried beneath layers of congested, confused, outdated emotions, thereby preventing natural elimination.

Reflexes

- See Nervous Disorders.
- Concentrate on the colon reflexes to ease the elimination of bodily wastes.

Other suggestions

- See Digestive Disorders.
- Spring-clean the house, office, school desk, etc.
- Flush out the body with fresh fruit juice and purified water for one or two days, followed by fresh fruit and vegetables only for a few days.
- Drink Black Forest tea to flush through system.
- A change of routine to discard old habits and ideas.

NAUSEA

Definition

Sensation of sickness with inclination to vomit.

Emotional aspect

Feeling uncomfortable and wanting to reject a situation or person.

Reflexes

- As for Digestive Disorders.
- Spend time on neck and shoulder reflexes to release the grip on the musculature.
- Digestive tract reflexes, concentrating on the stomach and liver reflexes, to ease peristalsis.

Other suggestions

- See Digestive Disorders.
- Sniff peppermint.
- Drink lemon balm herbal tea.
- Homoeopathic remedies: Ant. Crud. – for coated white tongue and loss of appetite; Apomorphia – for sudden nausea.

Footnote: *Challenging situations, no matter how unpalatable, can be used advantageously for inner growth and expansion by shifting the thought.*

PANCREAS

Definition

An endocrine and exocrine gland situated behind the stomach. It secretes pancreatic juices which ferment food particles in the duodenum and insulin secretions that balance blood sugar.

Emotional aspect

Eases the flow and sweetness of life.

Reflexes

- **Pancreatic reflexes**, immediately above the waistline on inner part of the insteps on both feet, for natural energy to enjoy all activities.

Characteristic reflexes

Swollen reflexes: indicate a craving for sweetness or chocolate, to substitute perceived lack of joy in life, or extreme hunger immediately before meals.
Sunken reflexes: have been temporarily drained of energy and enthusiasm.

Other suggestions

- Regular, small, nutritious energising meals.

Footnote: *There is joy in every aspect of life, only the amount differs and that alters with perception.*

PANCREATITIS

Definition

Inflammation of the pancreas.

Emotional aspect

Suppressed anger that erupts one to two years after an emotionally fraught circumstance that has robbed life of its sweetness and joy.

Reflexes

- Concentrate on the pancreatic reflexes for harmony and joy.
- Digestive reflexes to encourage the absorption of natural sweetness.

Other suggestions

- See Digestive Disorders.
- Eat wholesome, natural food, particularly fresh fruit, when craving sugar.

Footnote: *Do everything with love and love everything you do.*

PANCREAS

HYPOGLYCAEMIA

Definition

A lack of sugar/glucose in the blood.

Emotional aspect

Feeling overwhelmed and drained by the enormity of it all and consequently feeling that life lacks sweetness.

Reflexes

- As for Digestive Disorders.
- Concentrate on the pancreatic and liver reflexes for natural secretion, metabolism and distribution of sugar.

Other suggestions

- See Digestive Disorders.
- Eat regular small quantities of wholesome natural foods, preferably raw, for the continual release of energy.
- Enjoy fresh fruit for the immediate release of natural energy.

Footnote: *Joyful participation generates ongoing energy and enthusiasm for life.*

PEPTIC ULCER

Definition

Erosion of the stomach or duodenal mucous membrane due to
excessive acidity.

Gastric ulcer: on lesser curve of stomach.
Duodenal ulcer: on first part of duodenal tract.
Anastomatic ulcer: appears after surgery.

Emotional aspect

Eating away at the self. Feeling inadequate and not able to
please.

Reflexes

- As for Digestive Disorders.
- Digestive system reflexes, particularly the stomach and
  duodenal reflexes, to reduce acidity, pain, indigestion and
  flatulence so that self-esteem can be nourished. Concentrate
  on the cardiac sphincter reflexes to relieve heartburn.
- Liver reflexes to release feelings of inadequacy and
  frustration.

Other suggestions

- See Digestive Disorders.
- Relaxation techniques to relieve worry and anxiety.
- See Vomiting and Flatulence.
- Drink milk to neutralise excessive acidity.
- Eat bland, wholesome food, in small quantities, avoiding
  spices, fats, flavourings, pips, skins and alcohol.
- Homoeopathic remedies: Arsenicum – to ease severe,
  burning pain and exhaustion; Atropinum – to relieve severe
  mid-abdominal discomfort with nausea and vomiting;
  Ornithogalum – a general remedy; Nux vomica – to ease pain
  that is worse in the morning and is accompanied by
  irritability and headaches.

Footnote: *Life is the greatest possession of all – value it!*

PILES

See Haemorrhoids

SPASTIC COLON

Definition

Extreme muscular contraction causing sudden convulsive movement of the large colon.

Emotional aspect

Anger, fear or frustration at not being good enough. Pressure from driving the self due to unreasonably high expectations.

Reflexes

- As for Digestive Disorders.
- Spend time on digestive reflexes, concentrating on the colon and liver reflexes, for flexibility and adaptability.

Other suggestions

- See Digestive Disorders.
- Relaxation techniques for inner calm.

Footnote: *Everything done with unconditional love and joy is automatically rewarded with success.*

STOMACH DISORDERS

Definition

Interference with the harmonious expansion and contraction of the stomach, altered secretions or a change in the churning action prevent the natural breakdown of food for absorption.

Emotional aspect

Difficulty in breaking down ideas and experiences for personal growth and nourishment. Not 'stomaching' situations.

'Butterflies' in the stomach. Moods immediately affect stomach conditions:

During anger: blood rushes to the stomach lining, the outpouring of hydrochloric acid floods the sac and the churning movement becomes aggressive, destroying all nutrients in a subconscious attempt to escape the present situation by exterminating it.

During depression: the blood drains away from the stomach lining, the outpouring of hydrochloric acid is limited and churning becomes sluggish. A bloated feeling of being weighed down results due to disinterest or discontentment with present circumstances.

Reflexes

- As for Digestive Disorders.
- Central nervous system reflexes, concentrating on the brain, neck and solar plexus reflexes, for a more palatable outlook on life.
- Digestive reflexes, particularly the stomach and liver reflexes, to create a calm environment for natural digestion.
- Liver reflexes to release pent-up emotions.

Other suggestions

- See Digestive Disorders.
- Appreciate wholesome natural foods.
- Drink plenty purified fluids.
- Chew food well for easier digestion.

WORMS

Definition

Parasites that invade and inhabit the intestinal tract.

Tapeworm: A round head with suckers or hooks that attach themselves to the intestinal wall. Numerous segments grow and each segment is capable of producing ova that can survive independently for long periods.

Threadworm: tiny white worms found in faeces and around the anus.

Roundworms: ascaris lumbaricoides that also invade the bile duct, liver and trachea causing abdominal pain, diarrhoea or constipation.

Emotional aspect

Feeling victimised and invaded by the conflicting beliefs and attitudes of others that feed off and drain the self.

Reflexes

- As for Digestive Disorders.
- Spend time on the digestive system reflexes, concentrating on the intestinal reflexes, to ease the grip of the worms so that they can be expelled.

Other suggestions

- See Digestive Disorders.
- Massage both feet, especially the toes and insteps, with aromatherapy essential oils to assist with the elimination of worms: camomile, fennel, eucalyptus, grapefruit, lavender, lemon, tea-tree, thyme.

Footnote: *Be your own self and allow your individuality to colour the world with vibrancy.*

Skeletal and Muscular Systems

THE SKELETON

Definition

Hard, bony framework of dense connective tissue that contains and protects bodily organs.

Emotional aspect

Universal support and structure for physical, emotional, intellectual and spiritual mobility, flexibility, adaptability, growth and expansion.

Reflexes

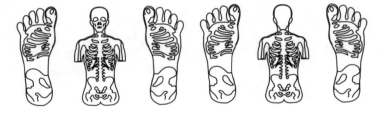

Anterior Skeletal reflexes - soles   *Posterior Skeletal reflexes - tops*

- **Skeletal reflexes** found throughout the feet, are massaged for inner strength, mobility and flexibility.
- **Head and toes**: protect and support thoughts and ideas.
- **Neck and shoulders**: allow for flexibility and mobility of expressions.
- **Upper torso, arms and legs**: support and embrace loving feelings.
- **Lower torso, arms and legs**: reinforce belief in and support activities.
- **Pelvic, hands, feet**: provide a foundation and basic security for expansion, growth and mobility.

Head and neck bone reflexes
Skull Bone reflexes, found on all toes, particularly on the nails, are massaged to protect ideas and create space for thought. They vibrate to purple/turquoise.

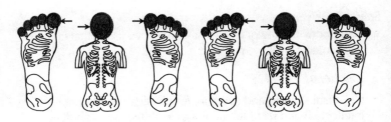

Anterior Skull reflexes - soles   *Posterior Skull reflexes - tops*

Neck Bone reflexes, found on the necks of all toes, are massaged for flexibility, adaptability and the free exchange of life's expressions. They vibrate to turquoise-blue.

Torso bone reflexes
Shoulder Bone reflexes found along the bases of all the little toes on the tops and on the soles of both feet, are massaged to lighten the load and carry messages of unconditional love, hope and joy. They vibrate to turquoise/blue.

Rib Bone reflexes, found on the hard balls and on the tops of both feet, are massaged to ease interaction within the

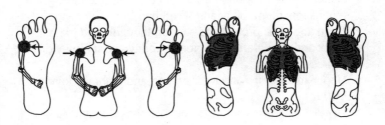

Shoulder reflexes   *Rib reflexes*

environment, and to generate feelings of well-being. They vibrate to turquoise/green.

Sternum Bone reflexes, found along the inner edges of the hard balls on both feet, are massaged to protect the soul and give it space for individuality. They vibrate to turquoise/green.

Spinal Bone reflexes are massaged for physical, emotional and spiritual support and security.

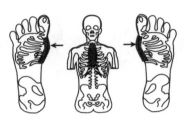

Sternum reflexes

Pelvic and Hip Bone reflexes, found on the balls of the heels and ankles of both feet, are massaged to provide enthusiasm and energy to thrust through life with confidence and joy. They vibrate to orange/red.

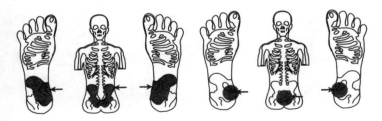

Pelvic reflexes   *Pubic bone reflexes*

Pubic Bone reflexes, found on the inner heels, are massaged to protect security and personal identity. They vibrate to red.

193

Arm reflexes

Upper Arm Bone reflexes, extend from the protruding bones immediately beneath the little toes, along the outer edges of both feet to the bony protuberances midway along the outer feet and are massaged to embrace life's expressions with love and joy. They vibrate to turquoise/green.

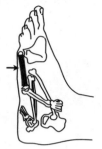

Upper arm bone reflexes

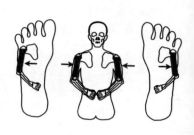

Upper arm reflexes

Elbow Bone reflexes are bony protrusions midway along the outer edges of both feet and are massaged for flexibility and the ability to adapt with ease to new situations. They also provide elbow room to experiment and venture along new avenues. They vibrate to green/yellow.

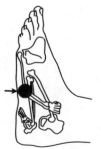

Elbow joint reflexes

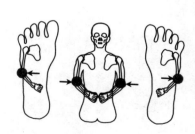

Elbow reflexes

Lower Arm Bone reflexes, from the elbow reflexes to swellings at the front of the outer ankle bones, are massaged to reach out to enjoy life's experiences. They vibrate to yellow/orange.

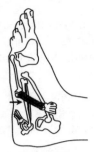

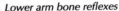
Lower arm bone reflexes

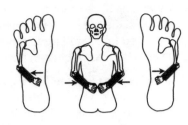
Lower arm reflexes

Wrist and Hand Bone reflexes are palpable swellings at the front of both ankle bones that are massaged to ease manipulation of life's details and to mould life's experiences with love and joy. They vibrate to red.

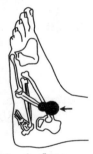

Wrist & hand reflexes

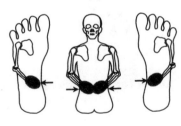

Wrist & hand reflexes

Finger Bone reflexes, found with the hand reflexes, are massaged for dexterity and the security of feeling at ease with the details of life. They vibrate to red.

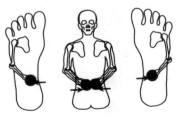

Finger reflexes

Leg reflexes

Upper Leg Bone reflexes extend from the base of the outer ankles to the knee (patella) reflexes, on both feet and are massaged for the full expression of life through freedom of movement. They vibrate to turquoise/green.

Knee (Patella) Bone reflexes situated fractionally above the midway point between shoulder and elbow reflexes and are massaged for increased flexibility and the natural control of movement. They vibrate to yellow.

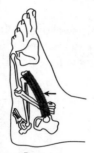

Upper leg reflexes

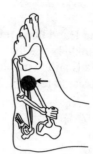

Knee bone reflexes

Lower Leg Bone reflexes follow from the knee reflexes, along the outer edges of both feet, to palpable swellings below outer ankle-bones. They vibrate to yellow.

Ankle bone reflexes, situated below the outer ankles on the outer edges of both feet, are massaged for flexibility and the ability to adapt to life's ups and downs. They vibrate to red.

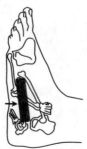

Lower leg reflexes

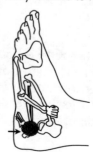

Ankle bone reflexes

Foot Bone reflexes, found on the outer edge of both feet, below the outer ankle-bones, are massaged to establish a firm footing and a secure base from which to step ahead with confidence and ease. They vibrate to red.

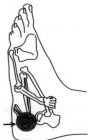

Foot bone reflexes

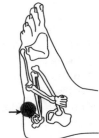

Toe bone reflexes

Toe Bone reflexes are part of the feet reflexes, and, like antennae, reach out for information to clarify the thought processes and to open the mind to the expansiveness of life's opportunities. They vibrate to red.

Characteristic reflexes

- An extra bone in the body is immediately reflected as an additional protusion in the applicable reflex on the foot.
- If a bone is missing or has been removed there is a corresponding gap in the foot.
- Crushed bone feels gritty in the related reflex on the foot.

Other suggestions

- Alexander Technique to realign the whole for inner strength and support.
- Check posture at all times.
- Bend knees to lift anything from a lower level.

SKELETAL DISORDERS

Definition

Interference with the skeletal substance, making bones rigid, weak or deformed.

Emotional aspect

Tension and anxiety impinge and erode the skeletal structure, stiffening it, weakening it and causing it to crumble.

Reflexes

- Concentrate on all the central nervous system reflexes, particularly the midbrain and solar plexus reflexes for expansion, agility and strength of mind.
- Neck and shoulder reflexes for the flexibility to adapt to all of life's expressions.
- Endocrine system reflexes, especially the pituitary, pineal, thymus and adrenal gland reflexes for inner strength and understanding.
- Chest reflexes to ease the interchange of internal and external life forces.
- Digestive system reflexes for growth and development, as well as fuel for movement.
- Liver reflexes to eliminate accumulated frustration.
- Arm and leg reflexes to release from the shackles of self constraint.
- Skeletal reflexes, concentrating on affected areas, for reinforcement of inner substances.
- Circulatory, lymphatic and urinary system reflexes to unload the body of unnecessary substances.
- All bodily reflexes (see foot chart) for inner support.

Other suggestions

- Professional guidance if required.
- Relaxation techniques to release mind, body and soul from the grips of fear and anxiety.
- Passive, pleasurable exercise to build up resources.
- Wholesome, natural food for inner strength.
- Vitamin and mineral supplements to revitalise the whole.
- If applicable, elevate and rest the affected part.
- Massage both feet, particularly the afflicted reflexes, as well as the affected bodily area, with aromatherapy oils.
  To accelerate healing: cypress, fennel, lavender, rosemary, thyme; to increase flexibility and mobility: cypress, camomile, carrot, ginger, hyssop, juniper; to ease muscular

spasm: hyssop, lavender, marjoram, rosemary; to reduce pain and ease pressure: camomile, eucalyptus, peppermint.
- Bach flower remedies to create space for the self.

MUSCULAR SYSTEM

Definition

Massive network of strong tissue composed of fibres that have amazing power to expand and contract, incredible strength and the ability to move bodily parts in co-ordination.

Emotional aspect

Ability to move through life with ease. Flexibility to adapt.

Reflexes

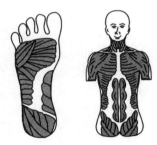
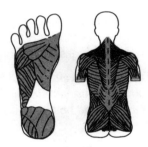

Anterior muscle reflexes - soles   *Posterior muscle reflexes - tops*

- **Muscular reflexes**, found throughout the feet, are massaged for adaptability and flexibility.
- **Head and toes**: mobilise and expand thoughts and ideas.
- **Neck and shoulders**: provide flexibility and mobility for the affirmation of expressions.
- **Upper torso, arms and legs**: allow expansive exchange of loving feelings.
- **Lower torso, arms and legs**: adapt to relationships and communicate with ease.

199

- **Pelvic, hands, feet**: provide power and mobility for expansive growth.

Head and neck muscle reflexes
Head Muscle reflexes, found on all toes, are massaged top and bottom for expansive thought. They vibrate to purple/turquoise.

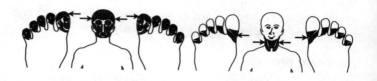

Head muscle reflexes   *Neck muscle reflexes*

Neck Muscle reflexes, found on the necks of all toes, are massaged for flexibility, adaptability and the free exchange of life's expressions. They vibrate to turquoise/blue.

Torso muscle reflexes
Shoulder Muscle reflexes, found along the bases of the little toes at the top and bottom of both feet, are massaged to facilitate the

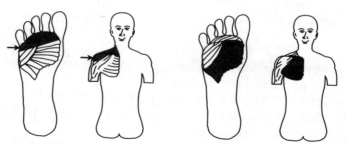

Shoulder muscle reflexes   *Intercostal muscle reflexes*

carrying of messages of unconditional love, hope and joy. They vibrate to turquoise/blue.

Intercostal Muscle reflexes, found on the hard balls and tops of both feet, are massaged to ease interaction within the environment and for feelings of well-being. They vibrate to turquoise/green.

Back Muscles reflexes are massaged for physical, emotional and spiritual support and security. They vibrate to all colours.

Pelvic and Hip Muscle reflexes, found on the heels and ankles of both feet are massaged to provide enthusiasm and energy to thrust through life with confidence and joy. They vibrate to orange/red.

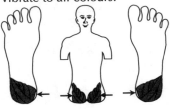

Pelvic & hip muscle reflexes

Arm reflexes

Upper Arm Muscle reflexes, from the protruding bones immediately beneath the little toes, along the outer edges of both feet to the bony protuberances midway along the outer feet, are massaged to embrace life's expressions with love and joy. They vibrate to turquoise/green.

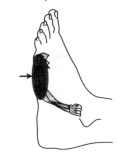

Upper arm muscle reflexes

Elbow Muscle reflexes are bony protrusions midway along the outer edges of both feet and are massaged for flexibility and the ability to adapt to new situations with ease and to provide elbow room to experiment and venture along new avenues. They vibrate to green/yellow.

Lower Arm Muscle reflexes, from the elbow reflexes to swellings to the front of outer ankle-bones, are massaged to reach out to enjoy life's experiences. They vibrate to yellow/orange.

Wrist and Hand Muscle reflexes are palpable swellings at the front of both ankle-bones and are massaged to ease

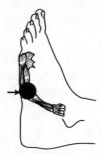

Elbow muscle reflexes

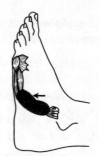

Lower arm muscle reflex

manipulation of life's details and to mould life's experiences with love and joy. They vibrate to orange/red.

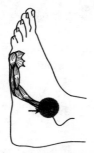

Wrist & hand muscle reflexes

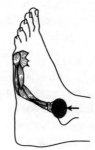

Finger reflexes

Finger Muscle reflexes, found with hand reflexes, are massaged for dexterity and security to feel at ease with the details of life. They vibrate to red.

Leg reflexes

Upper Leg Muscle reflexes, found from the base of the outer ankles to the knee (patella) reflexes on both feet, are massaged for the full expression of life through freedom of movement. They vibrate to turquoise/green.

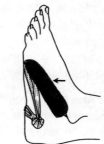

Upper leg muscle reflexes

Knee (Patella) Muscle reflexes, situated slightly above the midway point between the shoulder and elbow reflexes, are massaged for increased flexibility and the natural control of movement. They vibrate to yellow.

Lower Leg Muscle reflexes, follow from the knee reflexes, along outer edges of both feet, to swellings below outer ankles. They vibrate to orange/red.

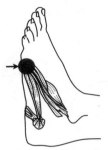

Knee (patella) muscle reflexes

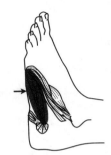

Lower leg muscle reflexes

Ankle Muscle reflexes, situated below the outer ankles on the outer edges of both feet are massaged for flexibility and the ability to adapt to life's ups and downs. They vibrate to orange/red.

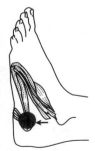

Ankle muscle reflexes

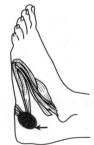

Foot muscle reflexes

Foot Muscle reflexes, found on outer edges of both feet, below the outer ankle-bones, are massaged to establish a firm footing and a secure base from which to step ahead with confidence and ease. They vibrate to red.

Toe Muscle reflexes are part of foot reflexes and are like antennae that reach out for information to clarify the thought process and open the mind to the expansiveness of life's opportunities. They vibrate to red.

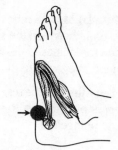

Toe muscle reflexes

ANKLE DISORDERS

Definition

Under duress the ankle joint is prone to:
Oedema;
Stretching or tearing of muscle;
Injury to ligament or;
Bone disorders.

Emotional aspect

Resistance to enjoyment and pleasures of life due to lack of inner security. Difficulty in adapting to life's ups and downs.

Reflexes

- As for Skeletal Disorders.
- Concentrate on the ankle reflexes for the free flow of life-forces to accelerate healing.

Other suggestions

- See Skeletal Disorders.
- Elevate and rest the affected ankle whenever possible.

ARM DISORDERS

Definition

Tension or injury inhibits the full movement and utilisation of the arms creating dis-ease.

Emotional aspect

Feeling that the wings have been clipped and that the arms are tied to the sides. Unable to embrace fully all of life's experiences. Fear of reaching out to keep in touch with natural process of life. Feeling unpleasantly out of control.

Reflexes

- As for Skeletal Disorders.

Other suggestions

- Allow the natural expression of life through creative activity.
- Freely move the arms to release rigidity.
- Lie on your back, open your arms, and breathe deeply.

ARTHRITIS

Osteo-Arthritis

Rheumatoid Arthritis

Pyogenic Arthritis

Definition

Inflammation of a joint.

> Osteoarthritis: extreme pain and restricted mobility from deterioration of the articular cartilage, aggravated by a diminished blood supply caused by tension.
> Rheumatoid arthritis: painful swollen joints and muscle-wasting from chronic inflammation of connective tissue. An imbalanced auto-immune system attacks healthy cells.
> Pyogenic arthritis: infection of a joint caused by a pyogenic organism.

Emotional aspect

Suppressed anger and frustration at having to conform to rigid belief systems, usually self-imposed, causing limitations of the body and mind. Generally perfectionists who believe everyone should have similar high standards.

Reflexes

- See Skeletal Disorders.
- Concentrate on all endocrine system reflexes, particularly the pituitary and adrenal gland reflexes, to reduce inflamed feelings.
- Reflexes of the affected areas (see foot chart), as well as reflexes of whole body, for overall ease and mobility.

Other suggestions

- See Nervous and Skeletal Disorders.
- The Arthritic Association, First Floor Suite, 2 Hyde Gardens, Eastbourne BN21 4PN.
- Seek professional guidance.
- See Nervous and Skeletal Disorders.
- Massage both feet with aromatherapy essential oils for increased flexibility and mobility: Osteoarthritis – basil, eucalyptus, lemon, ginger; Pyogenic arthritis – above, plus tea-tree; Rheumatoid arthritis – camomile, geranium, lavender, rosemary.
- Regular passive, but pleasurable, exercise mobilising the afflicted joints.
- Simplify household chores with handy, adapted gadgets.
- Herbal remedies: parsley, garlic, honeysuckle, feverfew.
- Bach flower remedies for increased tolerance of the self and others.
- Homoeopathic remedies: Rhus Tox. – basic remedy to use; Bryonia – to ease painful joints; Calc. Hypophos – to relax afflicted hands.
- Criticism is an adult's way of crying.

Footnote: *Variety and freedom openly create a more expansive and happier reality.*

BUNIONS

Definition

Inflammation and swelling of the metatarsal joint of the big toe, causing enlargement and deformity.

Emotional aspect

Anger at the self for conforming rigidly to a strictness that constrains mobility of thought. Inability to see other points of view. Common in perfectionists. Wanting to break away.

Reflexes

- As for Skeletal Disorders.

Gently massage the bunion as well as:

- Concentrate on the central nervous system reflexes, especially the solar plexus reflexes, to ease the pain and for mobility of thought.
- With regular reflexology the bunion can disappear as the big toe straightens.

Other suggestions

- See Skeletal Disorders.
- Although footwear is not the **cause**, it can certainly aggravate the situation. Walk barefoot whenever possible.
- Exercise the feet and stretch toes wide to expand the mind.
- Homoeopathic remedies: Hekla Lava – to reduce swelling; Agaricus – for irritability and redness.

BURSITIS

Housemaid's Knee

Dustman's Shoulder

Weaver's Bottom

Definition

Inflammation of the joint

Emotional aspect

Anger at having to restrain the self or from having progress and flexibility inhibited.

Reflexes

- As for Skeletal Disorders.
- Concentrate on the reflexes of affected joints to ease the discomfort.
- Circulatory, lymphatic and urinary system reflexes for the natural elimination of inflamed tissue and emotions.

Other suggestions

- See Skeletal Disorders.
- Apply an ice-pack for immediate relief.

Footnote: *Replace thoughts of desperation with love, joy and understanding.*

CRAMPS

Definition

Painful, involuntary, slow, forceful muscular contractions, often associated with muscle fatigue, dehydration or interference of toxic substances.

Emotional aspect

Undue tension and resistance in the muscles from intense fear and extreme anxiety.

Reflexes

- As for Skeletal Disorders.
- Spend time on the muscular reflexes, concentrating on the afflicted parts, to release from the grips of tension and allow the free exchange of life-forces.

Other suggestions

- During an attack hold both big toes and squeeze, applying firm pressure, top and bottom to reduce the discomfort.
- Vitamin and mineral supplements, particularly calcium, zinc and garlic capsules.

- Keep warm, especially cold feet. Place the feet under a pillow placed between sheets for added warmth.

Footnote: *Still the mind and release fearful, gripping thoughts.*

ELBOW DISORDERS

Definition

Pain and discomfort of the outer part of the joint between the forearm and upper arm.

Emotional aspect

Perceived need to elbow one's way through life. Resistance to a change of direction.

Reflexes

- As for Skeletal Disorders.
- Spend time on the arm reflexes, concentrating on the elbow reflexes, to release from the grips of anxiety, encourage flexibility, ease mobility and promote healing.

Other suggestions

- See Skeletal Disorders.
- Apply a heated flannel with a couple of drops of peppermint oil.

BACK

Definition

Physically supports and strengthens the body, mind and soul. Eases movement through life in an upright position.

Emotional aspect

Physical, emotional and spiritual backbone and support. The security provided allows for increased flexibility and adaptability.

209

Upper back: provides emotional strength.
Middle back: supports personal activities.
Lower back: provides a foundation and security upon which life is built.

Reflexes

- See Spinal Reflexes and massage for inner strength and basic security.

Other suggestions

- Check your posture at all times.
- The Alexander Technique realigns the body into its natural posture with a fair distribution of bodily weight so that all the muscles are at ease. The release and free flow of energy is incredibly rejuvenating. Society of Teachers of the Alexander Technique, 20 London House, 266 Fulham Road, London SW10 9EC. Tel: 0171-351 0828.
- Chiropractic manipulation: British Chiropractic Association, 29 Whitely Street, Reading, Berks RG2 0EG. Tel: 01734 757 557.
- Osteopathy: General Council of Osteopaths, 56 London Street, Reading, Berks RG1 4SQ. Tel: 01734 576 585.
- Relaxation techniques.

Footnote: *Universal strength comes from within.*

FEET

Definition

Relatively small bases that, with the legs, support the massive weight of the whole body. Incredibly flexible and mobile due to the numerous small bones, muscles and ligaments working in unison.

Emotional aspect

The basis of life and the foundation of all its experiences. Vital energy link between the body and the earth. Contact with the ground provides security to step ahead with joy and confidence. The spring in the step, or lack of it, indicates the amount of enthusiasm for life. Feet reflect an understanding of all aspects of life, as well as the relationship with the self and others.

Reflexes

- Massage feet reflexes to establish a firm footing and promote confidence to experience life to the full.

Other suggestions

- Foot baths with lavender oil to relax, and peppermint oil to cool.
- Regular pedicures. If feet look good, they feel good!
- Foot exercises: rotate ankles, stretch open toes, flex in all directions, and so on.
- Stretch the toes to create space to think!
- Walk in the open air and country, as often as possible, especially barefoot!
- Relaxation techniques.
- Modern dance for free expression of the true self.

Footnote: *Step ahead with love, joy and confidence to discover the wonders of life, adapting with ease to life's ups and downs.*

BACK DISORDERS

LUMBAGO

Definition

Lack of physical support, strength and flexibility.
Lumbago: girdle-like distribution of pain of lower back.

Emotional aspect

Perceived lack of support and security resulting in restricted mobility.
Upper back disorders: feelings and emotions receive no backing.

Middle back discomfort: remorse and regret regarding activities and communication.
Lower back pain: lack of security due to too great a dependence and concern with material aspects of life stunting personal development.

Reflexes

- Spend time on the central nervous system, concentrating on the spinal reflexes, for inner strength and flexibility of thought.
- Endocrine system, particularly the pituitary, pineal, thymus and adrenal gland reflexes, for emotional support.
- Back reflexes for adaptability and mobility.

Types of insteps

- See Spinal Disorders.

Other suggestions

- National Back Pain Association (NBPA), 16 Elmtree Road, Teddington, Middlesex TW11 8ST. Tel: 0181 977 5474/5.
- Relaxation techniques.
- Lie on your back with your legs bent, breathe deeply, smile and gently press the small of the back onto the floor. Allow the back time before it can lie completely flat.
- Check your posture at all times and keep the spine straight.
- Place your mattress on floor, or place on board.
- Bend your knees to pick up heavier objects.
- Meditation or other relaxation techniques for inner support and understanding.
- Alexander Technique, body alignment, acupuncture, osteopathy or chiropractic manipulation.
- Massage both feet, particularly the insteps, with aromatherapy essential oils for increased relief: camphor, camomile, juniper, lavender, rosemary.
- Bach flower remedies for encouragement and support.
- Homoeopathic remedies: Natrum Mur. – for relief from severe, chronic discomfort; Ruta – to ease lower back distress; Nux Vomica – to release nocturnal aches.

- During pregnancy, kneel on all fours to read and sit back to front on upright chairs to allow gravity to ease the pressure.

BREAKS AND FRACTURES

Definition

Direct or indirect violence that can break or fracture the bone, with extreme pain, swelling, deformity and loss of power. There is either restricted or no mobility.

Emotional aspect

Resistance to the natural flow of life and rebellion against a greater force or discipline causes bones to break or crack.

Reflexes

- As for Skeletal Disorders.
- All reflexes on both feet with particular attention to the affected bone reflexes (see foot chart) to ease the pain and increase the supply of essential nutrients for healing.

Other suggestions

- See Skeletal Disorders.
- Relaxation techniques for inner peace.

BONE DEFORMITY

Definition

Misplaced or mis-shapen bone.

Emotional aspect

A relaxed mind relaxes the body, facilitating freedom of expression and movement. Rigidity, from mental pressure and restrictive thinking, tightens the muscles causing a lack of mobility which stiffens and deforms bone.

Reflexes

- As for Skeletal Disorders.
- The reflexes of the afflicted area to release pressure and increase mobility.
- Lymphatic system reflexes to remove restrictions due to toxic accumulation.

Other suggestions

- See Skeletal Disorders.
- Massage both feet with aromatherapy essential oils to further relax the whole musculature: geranium, lavender, thyme.

FRACTURES

Definition

Broken bone accompanied by pain and swelling, either due to a direct or indirect impact.

Closed or simple fracture: clean break.

Comminuted fracture: several breaks.

Compound fracture: open fracture with skin damage.

Emotional aspect

Resisting or rebelling against the need to conform.

Reflexes

- As for Skeletal Disorders.
- Concentrate on the specific reflexes of the affected areas for new bone cell formation so that the bone can knit together.

Other suggestions

- See Skeletal Disorders.
- Use the time of restricted mobility constructively.
- Relaxation techniques for patience and understanding.
- Try to be as independent as possible.

Footnote: *The joys of life know no bounds and like to venture beyond the secure and tested pathways, for, only by testing the unknown, can new and exciting discoveries be made and enjoyed.*

FINGER DISORDERS

Definition

Pain or interference with functioning of digits on the hands.

Emotional aspect

Feeling that the hands are tied and restrained from moulding and manipulating the finer details of life due to fear or insecurity. Each digit is linked to a specific colour, bodily part or system and function. Disorders indicate:

Thumb: interference with intellectual, intuitive thoughts and ideas. Linked to the brain and central nervous system, vibrates to orange and has etherical qualities.

Index finger: feelings of self-esteem and self-worth are perceived to be battered or injured. Linked to the chest, particularly the heart and respiratory system, vibrates to yellow and has air qualities.

Middle finger: progress inhibited due to unresolved grudges and insecurity. Linked to the upper half of the digestive tract, especially the liver and stomach, vibrates to blue and has fire qualities.

Ring finger: painful communication and relationships, linked to the lower half of the digestive tract, as well as the urinary and circulatory system, vibrates to purple, and has water qualities.

Little finger: expansive thoughts and mobility of the mind restricted due to insecurity or the influence of upbringing. Linked to the skeletal system, especially the pelvis and limbs, vibrates to red and has earth qualities.

Unnatural reflexes

- Swollen or 'bruised' reflexes: frustration or pain at meeting resistance, especially when trying to deal with the little details in life. Feeling insecure because the hands feel tied and 'losing their grip'. Unable to 'keep in touch'!

Other suggestions

- See Hands.

FOOT DISORDERS

Definition

Unnatural afflictions of the feet.

Emotional aspect

Fear and frustration at what lies ahead and reluctance to step ahead. Feeling insecure because the 'rug has been pulled from under the feet'!

Reflexes

- As for Skeletal Disorders.
- Concentrate on the legs and feet reflexes for the strength and enthusiasm to stride ahead.

Other suggestions

- If severe, seek professional guidance.
  Massage both feet frequently with aromatherapy essential oils to further ease tension and increase mobility. Dancers – benzoin, geranium, tagetes, rosemary; Sportsmen – lavender, peppermint, rosemary, thyme.
- If swollen, soak the feet in iced water with three drops of lavender.
- For aches, soak the feet in warm water with three drops of rosemary and a teaspoon of baking powder.
- Regular pedicures. Feet that look good, feel good!

HAND DISORDERS

Definition

Interference with the natural activity and expression of the terminal part of the arms connected at the wrists.

Emotional aspect

Inability to handle, touch, feel, mould, manipulate or deal with life's experiences easily due to fear, insecurity and self-doubt.

Reflexes

- As for Skeletal Disorders.
- Concentrate on the hand reflexes for dexterity and freedom of expression. Swollen or discoloured (usually red or blue) reflexes indicate a feeling that the 'hands are tied' or are 'losing their touch'.

Other suggestions

- Exercise the hands, extending and flexing the digits.
- Massage both feet and the hands with aromatherapy essential oils to enhance freedom of movement and expression: geranium, jasmine, lavender, peppermint, rosemary, tagetes, thyme.
- Regular manicures. If hands look good they feel good.

Footnote: *Handle life's experience with excitement, anticipation and joy.*

HIP DISORDERS

Definition

Disorders and dis-eases of the hip due to tension causing the deprivation of essential life-forces and causing immobility.

Emotional aspect

Reluctance or fear of moving ahead.

Reflexes

- As for Skeletal Disorders.
- Spend time on the hip reflexes to release from the grips of fear and uncertainty.

Other suggestions

- Seek professional guidance. If severe, a hip replacement may be necessary.
- See Nervous and Skeletal Disorders.

HUNTINGTON'S CHOREA

See page 43 in The Nervous System section.

INGROWN TOENAIL

Definition

The toenails grow back into the skin.

Emotional aspect

Knocking the self and questioning one's own beliefs and ideas. Holding back because doubtful whether entitled to move ahead.

Reflexes

- As for Skeletal Disorders.
- Concentrate on the foot reflexes to ease tension and free the toenail.

Other suggestions

- See Skeletal Disorders.
- Seek professional guidance, particularly from a chiropodist.
- Regular pedicures to encourage the natural growth of the toenail.

Footnote: *Life is the soul's journey and, although souls travel together, each soul determines the best path for personal growth and enlightenment.*

JOINTS

Definition

Junction where two or more bones join together for flexibility and mobility.

Emotional aspect

Joints facilitate and ease changes of direction, physically, emotionally and spiritually.

Reflexes of mobile joints

Temporomandibular Joint, or Jaw reflexes found at bases of toe pads, are massaged for articulate ease. They vibrate to turquoise.

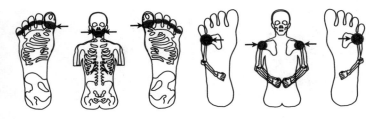

Temporomandibular joint/jaw reflexes   Shoulder reflexes

Shoulder Joint reflexes are palpable bony prominences below the little toes on the side to the top of the feet and are massaged for free expression and inner strength. They vibrate to green.

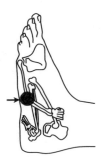 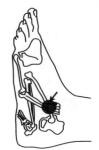

Elbow joint reflexes   Wrist joint reflexes

Elbow Joint reflexes are prominent projections of bone halfway along the outer edges of both feet and are massaged to accept openly the natural changes of life. They vibrate to yellow.

Wrist Joint reflexes are protruding bones at the bases of outer ankle-bones, on top of both feet and are massaged for joyful mobility. They vibrate to orange.

Finger Joint reflexes share the same reflexes as the wrists and are massaged for a secure base from which to expand. They vibrate to red.

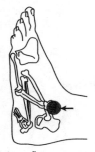

Finger joint reflexes

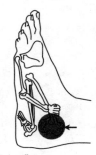

Hip joint reflexes

Hip Joint reflexes are found at the bases of the outer anklebones and are massaged to stride ahead with joy and confidence. They vibrate to turquoise.

Knee Joint reflexes. For the exact position place the thumbs on the bones below the little toes (shoulder reflexes) and the third fingers on protruding bone halfway along the outer edges of the feet (elbow reflexes), allowing the index fingers to rest midway, but slightly above. These reflexes are massaged for inner control through self-confidence and self-worth. They vibrate to green.

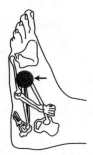

Knee joint reflexes

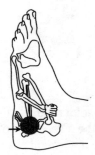

Ankle joint reflexes

Ankle Joint reflexes, situated immediately below the outer ankle-bones, on the lower, outer edges of the feet, and are massaged for the pleasure of being able to adapt to life's ups and downs with ease. They vibrate to orange.

Intervertebral Disc reflexes, found along the bony ridges on the inner aspects of both feet, are massaged for flexibility, mobility and security. They vibrate to red/orange/yellow/green/blue from the ankle to the neck of the big toe.

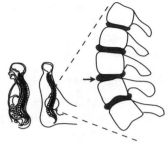

Intervertebral disc reflexes

Characteristic reflexes

- Swollen or protruding reflexes: resisting a change in direction.
- Red reflexes: angry or embarrassed about changes.
- Hard skin over reflexes: protecting decisions to change course or protecting the self from having to change.

Other suggestions

- Relaxation techniques for inner strength and flexibility.
- Exercise for pleasure rather than to compete. Games should be **fun**!

Footnote: Move with ease and adapt to the exciting changes in life with love and joy.

JOINT DISORDERS

Definition

Pain and discomfort in a joint.

Emotional aspect

Resistance to bending and changing to adapt to new circumstances.

Reflexes

- As for Skeletal Disorders.
- Give extra attention to the specific joint reflexes to facilitate movement.
- All bodily reflexes on both feet to relax the whole and for overall flexibility.

Other suggestions

- See Skeletal Disorders.
- Resistance creates pain, so go with the flow and allow fluidity of movements.
- Rest and apply ice to the affected joint initially, then later apply heat, a compress and elevate.
- Homoeopathic remedies: Bryonia – for discomfort that worsens with mobility; Rhus Tox – for stiffness and discomfort that ease with movement; Ruta – useful for painful hip and larger joints; Synovitis – to ease inflamed joints.

KNEE DISORDERS

Definition

Inefficient, disjointed activity and mobility of the knee joint.

Emotional aspect

Unable to move ahead with confidence and ease.

Reflexes

- As for Skeletal Disorders.
- Concentrate on the neck, shoulder, leg and knee reflexes to increase flexibility and step ahead with pride and joy.
- Liver reflexes to release overinflated opinions.

Other suggestions

- See Skeletal Disorders.
- Massage both feet, especially the knee reflexes, with aromatherapy essential oils to further encourage the release from the grips of tension: clove, ginger, nutmeg.

LEG DISORDERS

Definition

Interference with the legs' ability to support and mobilise.

Emotional aspect

Walking is an outward expression of inner emotions and feelings. The eager have a spring in their step, whilst the disinterested, disillusioned and fearful shuffle their way through life. Disorders indicate a reluctance or fear to move on, physically, emotionally, intellectually or spiritually.

Reflexes

- As for Skeletal Disorders.
- Concentrate on the leg reflexes to strengthen and facilitate mobility.
- All bodily reflexes on both feet for overall harmony and a balanced approach to life.

Other suggestions

- See Skeletal Disorders.
- Rest with the feet elevated.
- Regular pedicures for a comfortable base to step ahead.

MULTIPLE SCLEROSIS

Definition

Hardening of any part, particularly the muscle, from the excessive growth of fibrous and connective tissues.

Emotional aspect

Deep fear hardens thoughts and emotions to protect the self.

Reflexes

- As for Skeletal Disorders.
- Spend time on liver, circulatory, lymphatic and urinary system reflexes to free the whole of unnecessary encumbrances.

- Reflexes of the affected areas (see the foot chart) to release the grip on the musculature and to create space for flexibility and healing.

Other suggestions

- See Skeletal and Nervous Disorders.
- Inform the local health visitor and social worker.
- The Multiple Sclerosis Society of Great Britain and Northern Ireland, 25 Effie Road, London SW6 1EE.

MUSCULAR DISORDERS

Definition

Tension creates discomfort of the strong contractile fibrous bands or bundles interfering with movement and mobility. An ineffective nerve supply causes profound weakness and muscle wasting.

Emotional aspect

Reluctance to move ahead due to fear, anxiety, frustration and disappointment creating a resistance to the natural flow of life.

Reflexes

- As for Skeletal Disorders.
- Concentrate on lymphatic system reflexes to lighten the load and make space for fluidity of movement.
- Reflexes of the affected areas (see the foot chart) for increased mobility.

Other suggestions

- See Skeletal and Nervous Disorders.

MUSCULAR DYSTROPHIES

Definition

Progressive muscle wastage due to an ineffective nerve supply. Profound weakness. If wasted muscle is replaced with fat it looks larger than it should and is known as pseudo-hypertrophic muscle.

Emotional aspect

Self-restriction due to a deep fear, a lack of confidence or reluctance to move ahead and grow with ease.

Reflexes

- As for Skeletal Disorders.
- Spend time on the limb reflexes to strengthen muscles and improve the characteristic waddling gait.
- All bodily reflexes on both feet for inner strength and determination to move ahead with confidence and joy.

Other suggestions

- See Skeletal and Nervous Disorders.
- Muscular Dystrophy Group, 7–11 Prescott Place, Clapham, London SW4 6BS. Tel: 0171-720 8055.
- Massage both feet with aromatherapy essential oils to further strengthen the muscles. To stimulate – basil, eucalyptus, ginger, rosemary. To relax – geranium, lemon, orange, palma rose.
- Natural, wholesome food avoiding preservatives, colourants and additives to build up your resources.
- Supplement vitamin and mineral intake to boost vitality.
- Fill life with laughter and joy to slow down the degeneration.

Footnote: *Love of life provides the fuel and enthusiasm to spurt the whole into joyful action!*

OSTEOMYELITIS

Definition

Acute inflammation of the bone and its marrow.

Emotional aspect

Anger and frustration with lack of structural support in life.

Reflexes

- As for Skeletal Disorders.
- Concentrate on all bone reflexes for inner strength and understanding.
- All skeletal reflexes on both feet for overall support.

Other suggestions

- See Skeletal Disorders.
- Avoid carrying heavy loads.
- Wholesome, nutritious food to build up structural support.
- Vitamin and mineral supplements to boost enthusiasm.
- Drink plenty of purified fluids to flush through inflammation.
- Nettle tea or broth.
- Mild exercise to stimulate bone marrow formation.

OSTEOPOROSIS

Definition

Lack of mineral salts in the bones due to deficiency either of proteins or hormones in the bony matrix.

Emotional aspect

Feeling unsupported.

Reflexes

- See Osteomyelitis.

Other suggestions

- See Osteomyelitis.

PAGET'S DISEASE

Definition

Dense bone formation due to the overactivity of osteoblasts and osteoclasts.

Emotional aspect

Overcompensating because no one seems concerned and therefore there is no perceivable support to rely on.

Reflexes

- Central nervous system reflexes, concentrating on all reflexes, for a shift in perceptions and to prevent a curvature of the spine, and the skull bone from thickening.
- Endocrine system reflexes, particularly the pituitary, pineal, thyroid and thymus gland reflexes, for emotional strength.
- Bone reflexes to naturalise the bone cell formation.
- Leg reflexes to strengthen and prevent from bowing.
- Lymphatic system reflexes to eliminate the excessive number of osteoblasts and osteoclasts.
- All bodily reflexes on both feet to balance the body, mind and soul.

Other suggestions

- See Bone Deformities and Skeletal Disorders.

REPETITIVE STRAIN STRESS (RSS)/INJURY (RSI)/DISORDER (RSD)

TENNIS ELBOW

WRITER'S CRAMP

Definition

Pain, inflammation and stiffness of the soft tissue, muscles, tendons or ligaments due to ongoing tension from repetitive action. Common amongst musicians and dancers.

Emotional aspect

Determination to be in control.

Reflexes

- The reflexology massage relaxes first the physical body and then eases the mind, allowing for a more relaxed approach to life.

- Central nervous system, especially the midbrain and solar plexus reflexes, to calm nerves, ease pain, numbness, tingling and stiffness, as well as to make space for the natural subconscious control of muscles, tendons and ligaments.
- Endocrine system reflexes, particularly the pituitary, pineal, thymus and adrenal gland reflexes, to reduce inflammation and tenderness, and for inner peace.
- Muscular and skeletal system reflexes, concentrating on the neck, shoulder and affected reflexes, to ease the grip on the musculature so that the muscular swelling can reduce and natural mobility be reinstated.
- Circulatory, lymphatic and urinary reflexes for the free flow of essential life-forces and on-going elimination of toxic substances.

Other suggestions

- See Skeletal Disorders.
- Rest to ease the strain.
- Place ice-packs made up with loosely crushed ice on the affected area.

Footnote: *Trust universal guidance for true control.*

RHEUMATISM

Definition

Inflammation of the sheaths of muscles and joints, with acute pain, swelling and stiffness of one or more joints.

Emotional aspect

Anger and resentment at social restrictions and the need to conform to rigid belief systems that threaten personal identity and security.

Reflexes

- As for Skeletal Disorders.
- Concentrate on the reflexes of the affected areas (see foot

chart) to release from the grips of tension and to accelerate healing.
• All bodily reflexes (see foot chart) to facilitate mobility.

Other suggestions

• See Skeletal Disorders.
• Inform the local health visitor and social worker if incapacitated.
• Ease mobility with aids.
• Passive aqua exercises to strengthen the whole.
• Herbal remedies: Apple herb tea; Nettle herb tea; Rosemary herb tea.

Footnote: *Freedom of choice comes with true acceptance and unconditional love of the self.*

RHEUMATOID ARTHRITIS

Definition

Progressive incapacitating disease due to chronic inflammation of the fibrous connective tissue around the joints. Excruciating pain and increasing disabilities.

Emotional aspect

Anger at having movements inhibited by the authority of others.

Reflexes

• As for Skeletal Disorders.
• Concentrate on the reflexes of the affected areas (see foot chart) to nurture and promote healing.
• All bodily reflexes (see foot chart) for mobility and flexibility.

Other suggestions

• See Rheumatism.

Footnote: *No one and nothing is a threat unless allowed to be.*

RICKETS

Definition

Lack of vitamin D, especially in young babies and children,
preventing the absorption of phosphorus and calcium in the body.

Emotional aspect

Perceived lack of emotional love, support and security.

Reflexes

- As for Skeletal Disorders.
- Spend time on the circulatory and heart reflexes for the free
  distribution of love and joy.
- Reflexes of the affected areas (see foot chart) to nurture and
  support the healing process.

Other suggestions

- See Bone Deformity and Skeletal Disorders.

Footnote: *Look within and open up to universal strength for the
courage to step ahead with love and joy.*

ROUND SHOULDERS

Definition

Collapse of stature due to the shoulders folding forwards.

Emotional aspect

Bearing too much weight on the shoulders. Weighed down from
taking on and carrying perceived burdens and responsibilities
alone.

Reflexes

- As for Skeletal Disorders.
- Spend time on the shoulder reflexes to ease the load.
- Circulatory, lymphatic and urinary system reflexes to remove
  unnecessary burdens.

Other suggestions

- See Back and Skeletal Disorders.

Footnote: *Every situation is a challenge to discover more about the self and the world around us.*

SCOLIOSIS

LORDOSIS

KYPHOSES

Definition

Curvature of the spine.
    Scoliosis: usually a lateral deviation.
    Kyphosis: a humpback with posterior curvature of the spine.
    Lordosis: an unnatural forward curve of the lumbar spine.

Emotional aspect

Little or no belief in universal support and succumbing to social pressures and belief systems.

Reflexes

- See Spinal Reflexes and Skeletal Disorders.

Other suggestions

- See Spinal Reflexes and Skeletal Disorders.

Footnote: *Trust the natural process of life to provide inner strength, support and knowledge at all times.*

SPASMS

SPASTICITY

Definition

Extreme muscular contraction causing sudden convulsive movement.

Emotional aspect

Intense fear taking hold and gripping the body.

Reflexes

- As for Skeletal Disorders.
- Concentrate on the muscular reflexes, especially the affected areas, for flexibility and adaptability.

Other suggestions

- See Skeletal Disorders.
- Inform the local authorities, health visitor and social worker.
- Scope, 12 Park Crescent, London W1N 4EQ.

SPINE

Definition

The backbone or vertebral column that supports the body and keeps it upright. It also protects the spinal cord.

Emotional aspect

Provides support and the sensitivity to adapt to life's ups and downs.

Reflexes

- See page 000.

Other suggestions

- Alexander Technique to realign the whole.
- Check posture at all times.
- Relaxation techniques to enhance strength and sensitivity.

SPRAIN

Definition

Violent twist of a joint causing laceration, stretching, tearing or overextending of ligaments, with swelling and fluid effusion into the affected part.

Emotional aspect

Resistance and anger at having to adapt and move in a particular direction.

Reflexes

- As for Skeletal Disorders.
- Spend time on the specific reflexes to nurture, balance and promote healing.

Other suggestions

- See Skeletal Disorders.

STIFF NECK

Definition

Rigid rotation of the bodily part that connects the head and shoulders. Little or no flexibility of the neck.

Emotional aspect

A pain in the neck! Rigidity of thought arising from extreme fear and insecurity.

Difficulty in turning to right: not wanting to see something in the past.

Difficulty in turning to left: not wanting to see something in the future.

Difficulty in turning either way: stuck in a self-constructed rut with blinkers firmly in place!

Reflexes

- As for Skeletal Disorders.
- Reflexology eases neck stiffness with partial or complete return of flexibility within the hour!
- Toe pull and rotation for increased flexibility.
- Achilles stretch to expand the whole.
- Concentrate on the neck and throat reflexes to break away from rigid concepts.

Other suggestions

- See Skeletal Disorders.
- Ice-pack or heat further relieve discomfort.
- Chiropractic manipulation to further increase mobility, if required.

TEMPOROMANDIBULAR JOINT

See Jaw Disorders

TETANUS AND TETANY

See also Lockjaw

Definition

An anaerobe, clostridium tetani, found in the soil, that enters and infects the body through wounds, causing muscle rigidity particularly of the face and jaw.

Tetany: increased excitability of the nerves, due to a lack of calcium, causing painful muscular contraction.

Emotional aspect

Harbouring revengeful thoughts.

Reflexes

- As for Skeletal Disorders.
- Concentrate on all central nervous system reflexes, for expansion of the mind to release revengeful thoughts.
- Concentrate on the face, jaw and shoulder reflexes to relax muscular rigidity.

Other suggestions

- See Skeletal Disorders.
- Spring-clean the house, office, desk, etc. to release the old on all levels.
- Drink plenty of nutritious fluids if it is difficult to eat.

TICS

Twitches

Definition

Spasmodic contraction of a particular muscle, especially facial muscles.

Emotional aspect

Deep anxiety at having to face certain situations under the scrutiny of others.

Reflexes

- As for Skeletal Disorders.
- Concentrate on the central nervous system reflexes for the strength of mind to face any situation.

Other suggestions

- See Skeletal Disorders.
- Bach flower remedies, particularly Rescue Remedy during times of extreme anxiety.

TOES

Definition

Digits on feet.

Emotional aspect

Toes reflect thoughts and perceptions.
  Upstanding, well spaced toes with slight gaps between them: indicate open-mindedness.
  Bent toes: indicate conformity to other belief systems.
  Crushed toes: are indicative of having no space to think.

Reflexes

- Toe reflexes for flexibility and adaptability.

Other suggestions

- Regular creams and pedicures. Toes that look good, feel good!
- Foot baths.
- Enjoyable exercise to keep you on your toes!
- Stretch toes wide apart – especially when anxious.

Footnote: *From time to time, stop and go on tip-toes to see the pleasures and joys of life.*

WISDOM TEETH

Impacted

See Head, Neck and Sensory Organs

*r*EPRODUCTIVE SYSTEM

REPRODUCTIVE GLANDS AND ORGANS

Definition

Communication with life through procreation to produce lovingly new individuals on the pattern of existing ones.

Emotional aspect

An innate need for mankind to make sure that the cycle of evolution continues.

Reflexes

Male reproductive organs and glands
Penis reflexes, found on the inner heels, below the inner ankle-bones, are massaged for the natural ejaculation of sperm, and to ease the flow of urine and vibrate to red.

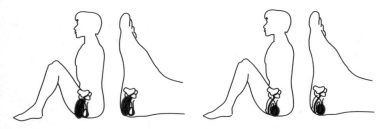

Penis reflexes   Testes reflexes

Testicle reflexes are palpable swellings on the inner heels, below the inner ankle-bones and are massaged for the natural production and secretion of healthy sperm. Due to the mobility of the testes, these reflexes are mobile on the feet and vibrate to red.

Prostate Gland reflexes, situated near the hollows midway between the tips of the heels and the inner ankle-bones, are massaged to allow active involvement in the reproductive cycle. They vibrate to red.

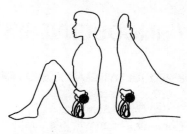

Prostate reflexes

Female reproductive organs Vagina and Cervix reflexes, situated on the hollows midway between the tips of the heels and the inner ankle-bones, with the remainder of the vaginal and cervix reflexes stretching from those points, and are massaged to enhance feminity. They vibrate to red.

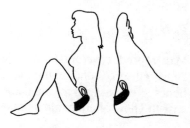

Vaginal reflexes

Uterine reflexes, found on the lower fleshy insteps, as well as on the sides of both feet, next to the distinctive mounds, are massaged to nurture and prepare for possible pregnancy. They vibrate to red/orange.

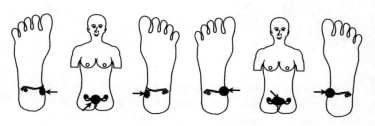

Uterine reflexes   *Uterus reflexes*

Characteristic Uterine Reflexes

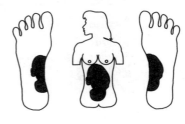

- See also Pregnant Uterine Reflexes.

- Swollen reflexes at any other time indicate a need to protect the feminine principle.

Pregnant reflexes

- Broken superficial blood vessels on these reflexes suggest perceived emotional or physical abuse or that feminity is being taken advantage of.

Fallopian Tube and Fallopian Finger reflexes, found on the soles, can also be massaged along their secondary accesses over the ankle creases on the tops of both feet, to be kept patent and viable. They vibrate to red/orange.

Characteristic Fallopian Tube reflexes

- The path of the ova along the tubes can be detected through the movement of a minute swelling over one of the ankle creases during alternate months.

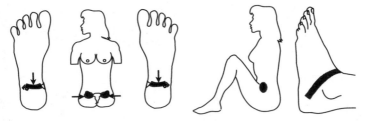

Fallopian tube & finger reflexes   *Fallopian tube & finger reflexes*

Ovary reflexes, found on the lower edges towards the outer parts of the fleshy insteps, have secondary accesses on the outer hollows, between the tips of the heel and the outer ankle-bones. They are massaged for the creation of new energy and vibrancy. They vibrate to red/orange.

Characteristics of Ovary reflexes

- These hollows can be very sensitive since they also reflect the indentations above the buttocks, which tend to accumulate tension, and are also known as 'high stress areas'.

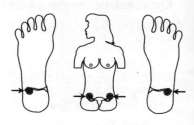

Ovary reflexes

- Alternate ovulation of the ovaries is reflected on the feet by the ovulating ovary reflex swelling considerably prior to ovulation whilst the other ovary reflex is hardly palpable. After ovulation the ovulating ovary reflex temporarily disappears.

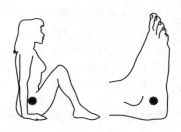

Ovaries reflexes

- During menstruation, both ovary reflexes are equally vibrant.
- The contraceptive pill inhibits ovulation and can likewise reduce the vibrancy and swelling of ovary reflexes.
- Concentrate on these reflexes: if ovaries have been removed, for irregular menstruation, during and after the menopause, or prior to the menarche (onset of menstruation).

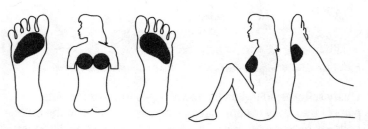

Breast reflexes   *Breast reflexes*

Breast reflexes are mounds on the hard balls of both feet and are massaged for the natural nurturing and nourishment of the self and others. They vibrate to green.

There are male and female characteristics in every person, so all above reflexes should be massaged regardless of gender for balance.

Other suggestions

- Women's Health, 52–54 Featherstone Street, London EC1Y 8RT.
- National Childbirth Trust, Alexander House, Oldham Terrace, Acton, London W3 6NH. Tel: 081-992 8637
- Regular check-ups.

REPRODUCTIVE AND GENITAL DISORDERS

Definition

Discomfort or dis-ease of the organs of procreation.

Emotional aspect

Dissatisfaction or discomfort with male or female characteristics. Concern about being inadequate.

Reflexes

Both partners should be treated. See also Gynaecological Disorders

- Central nervous system reflexes, especially the big, fourth and fifth toes, to shift ideas and concepts of self.
- Endocrine reflexes, concentrating on all gland reflexes, for emotional well-being and identification with true self.
- Digestive system reflexes to nurture the whole.
- Liver reflexes for inner calm.
- Circulatory, lymphatic and urinary system reflexes to drain away hampering ideas and replenish with fresh, creative thoughts.

- Female or male reproductive organ reflexes for ease with sexual characteristics.
- Urinary system reflexes, specifically urethral reflexes, to ease urination, if applicable.
- All bodily reflexes to project a favourable image.

Other suggestions

- Seek professional guidance.
- Massage both feet, concentrating on the toes, heels and insteps, with aromatherapy essential oils to further enhance self-identity: jasmine, neroli, patchouli, rose, rosewood, sandalwood, vetiver.
- To enhance sexuality: camomile, cypress, fennel, geranium, jasmine, neroli, rose, sandalwood, patchouli, ylang-ylang, vertivert. For inner peace: clary sage, cypress, geranium, nutmeg, rose. To accelerate healing: carrot, clove, cyprus, frankincense, lavender, lemon, myrrh, rose. For infections: tea tree.
- Vitamin and mineral supplements for increased vitality and fortification.
- Relaxation techniques to make space for the self and for inner calm.
- To look good is to feel good, so take pride in personal hygiene, appearance and dress according to gender.
- Bach flower remedies for improved self-confidence, self-acceptance and self restraint.

AMENORRHOEA

Definition

Absence of menstruation due to lack of maturity, pregnancy, menopause or disease.

Emotional aspect

Unnatural amenorrhoea arises from a subconscious denial of the female energy due to poor self-image or from extreme frustration at being a female in a male-dominant environment.

Reflexes

- As for Reproductive and Gynaecological Disorders.
- Concentrate on all central nervous system reflexes to boost self-confidence and release frustration.
- Female reproductive organ reflexes for naturally creative female energies.

Other suggestions

- See Reproductive Disorders.
- Homoeopathic remedies: Natrum Mur. – to increase, speed up or promote menstruation; Pulsatilla – to regulate menstruation; Sepia – to boost self-esteem; Sulphur – to naturalise menstruation.

BREAST

Definition

Female mammary gland that nurtures and suckles offspring.

Emotional aspect

Characteristic aspects of the breasts depend on perceptions of self-nourishment and the perceived need to nourish others.

Reflexes

- **Breast reflexes** found on the hard balls of both feet are massaged to release tension and supply the mammary cells with the natural amount of nourishment and nurturing.
- Breast reflexes overlap the chest reflexes symbolising that feelings about the self depend on self-nurturing and upbringing. The resulting degree of self-confidence and self-esteem directly influences the nature of interaction within the environment. Good feelings about the self allows for ease of interaction no matter what the circumstances.

Characteristic reflexes

- Lumpy reflexes: hide intense feelings about demanding people or situations within the environment.

- Taut, flattened reflexes: a feeling of being strained and worn out.
- Insteps impinge on the balls of the feet: perception that others are invading self-appointed territories.
- Blisters, shiny skin: heartfelt friction and hurt feelings; rubbing up against others.
- Flaking skin: irritability and conflict within the environment. Being rubbed up the wrong way!
- Plantar warts: frustration at the basis of self-understanding.
- Hard skin on balls of feet: protects feelings of self-esteem and self-worth. Trying to make space for the self, especially if nurturing others.
- Swollen, protruding bone on either side of the balls of the feet: feeling that the arms are tied with no room for expansive feelings and emotions.

Footnote: *Love and nurture the self and allow others to nurture themselves.*

BREAST DISORDERS

Definition

Tension inhibits the natural development of breast tissue. Mammary cells deprived of essential nutrients are prevented from functioning naturally.

Emotional aspect

Lumps, cysts and painful breasts contain pockets of congested emotions and feelings. Inflammatory disorders arise from festering anger and frustration regarding the maternal aspects of life.

Reflexes

- Concentrate on all central nervous system, particularly the solar plexus reflexes, for mental tranquillity.
- All endocrine system reflexes for emotional calm, inner peace and understanding.

- Neck and shoulder reflexes to allow for the full expansion of the chest.
- Breast reflexes for self-nurturing.
- Liver reflexes to release pent-up anger and resentment.
- Circulatory, lymphatic and urinary reflexes for the free flow of essential life-forces and the elimination of all toxic substances.
- All bodily reflexes for overall nurturing.

Other suggestions

- Iron a cabbage leaf and place inside the brassière over the affected breast, to relieve discomfort and inflammation. Especially good for nursing mothers.
- Massage both feet, especially the hard balls, with aromatherapy essential oils to promote healing.

Footnote: *Care for the self, to have the strength to encourage others to help themselves!*

ENDOMETRIOSIS

Definition

Excessive activity of womb lining. Rogue endometrial cells, which normally line the uterus, travel to other parts of the pelvis and body.

Emotional aspect

Thicker lining provides extra protection for feminity against abuse, disillusionment, frustration and fear.

Reflexes

- As for Reproductive and Gynaecological Disorders.
- Spend time on the female reproductive system reflexes, concentrating on the uterus reflexes, to release from the grips of anxiety so that the extra lining can be expelled and natural functioning can take place.
- All affected reflexes (see foot chart) to make space for the rogue cells to be absorbed and for natural cells to form.

Other suggestions

- See Reproductive Disorders.
- Vitamin and mineral supplements for increased vitality and fortification.

Footnote: *Female energy is in perfect synchronisation with natural life-forces and is powerful enough to heal, cherish and recreate mankind lovingly.*

FIBROID TUMOURS AND CYSTS

Fibromyoma

Definition

The unnatural swelling of fibrous and muscular tissue particularly in the uterus.

Emotional aspect

Accumulated resentment due to emotional hurts to the female ego.

Reflexes

- As for Reproductive and Gynaecological Disorders
- Concentrate on the brain reflexes, to release tension and calm demoralising mind talk.
- Female reproductive system, especially the uterus reflexes, to ease swelling, discomfort, reduce menses loss and create a favourable healing environment.

Other suggestions

- See Reproductive Disorders.
- Homoeopathic remedies: Aurum Mur – a useful long-term remedy; Calc. iodine – the best basic remedy; Sepia – to relieve the 'bearing down' discomfort.

Footnote: *Self-confidence promotes unconditional love for the self and for others.*

FRIGIDITY

Definition

Inability to respond lovingly and participate in natural sexual ardour and intimacy.

Emotional aspect

Emotions arising from a fear of masculine power.

Reflexes

- As for Reproductive and Gynaecological Disorders.
- Spend time on female reproductive organ reflexes to feel at ease with feminity.
- All bodily reflexes to open the self to the love and joy of sharing and being part of the whole

Other suggestions

- See Reproductive Disorders.
- Massage both feet, particularly the toes, heels and instep, with aromatherapy essential oils to heighten awareness of sensuality: bergamot, frankincense, geranium, jasmine, rose, ylang-ylang.
- Exercise the pelvic floor muscles.
- Feel at ease with sexual partner. Bathe together with one or more of above essential oils added to the water, with romantic music in the background, candlelight, champagne and afterwards lovingly caress each other.

Footnote: *Enjoy the gift of love and the joys of intimacy.*

GENITAL WARTS

Definition

Harmless, soft skin projections that flourish in the warm, moist environments, in and around the entrance of the vagina in females, or under the foreskin, on the shaft of the penis, or on the scrotum in males.

Emotional aspect

Small eruptions directed towards the sexual partner, or projections of guilt about one's own sexuality.

Reflexes

- As for Reproductive Disorders.
- Concentrate on the central nervous system reflexes, especially the big, fourth and fifth toes, for mobility of thought into realms of self-acceptance.

Other suggestions

- See Reproductive Disorders.
- Regular check-ups.
- Use condoms, lubricants, and make love gently to avoid abrasions.
- Apply directly to warts: Tea-tree essential oil; dandelion sap; crushed garlic in lemon or castor oil!

Footnote: *Look for the beauty within.*

GONORRHOEA

Definition

Venereal disease from intercourse or physical contact with gonococcal infection causing acute, purulent inflammation of the genital tract.

Emotional aspect

Personal disatisfaction due to lack of self-worth and respect.

Reflexes

- Central nervous system reflexes, especially the big, fourth and little toes, to raise level of consciousness and feelings of self-worth.
- Concentrate on the eye reflexes to reduce possible iritis or conjunctivitis.

- Endocrine system reflexes, particularly the pituitary, pineal, thymus and adrenal gland reflexes, for inner harmony and emotional security.
- Circulatory system reflexes to reduce infection within the blood and to prevent the spread of the infection.
- Lymphatic and urinary reflexes, concentrating on the ureteral reflexes, to eliminate toxic substances, to expand strictures and to reduce purulent discharge.
- Reproductive system reflexes to reduce discomfort, enhance blood supply and accelerate recovery.

Other suggestions

- See Reproductive Disorders.
- Seek professional guidance. Gonorrhoea responds well to antibiotics.
- Massage both feet, particularly the toes, heels and insteps with aromatherapy essential oils to further reduce inflammation: cinnamon, clove, eucalyptus, garlic, lemon, tea-tree, thyme.
- Nettle herb tea or broth to ease irritation.
- Personal hygiene to cleanse the self.
- Nourishing, wholesome food to build up resistance.
- Plenty of purified fluids, especially water, to flush through toxic substances.

Footnote: *Release mind, body and soul from the shackles of unreasonable expectations.*

GYNAECOLOGICAL DISORDERS

Definition

Diseases related to the female reproductive system, such as menstrual disorders and fibroid growths.

Emotional aspect

Discontent, discomfort or frustration with being a female, particularly in male-dominant situations where females are perceived to be the weaker sex.

Reflexes

- See also Reproductive Disorders.
- Central nervous system reflexes, especially the solar plexus reflexes, to boost self-confidence and reduce the level of frustration.
- Endocrine system reflexes for emotional control, personal space and the favourable enhancement of feminity.
- Female reproductive organ reflexes, particularly of affected parts, to release muscular tension and renourish the whole.
- Circulatory, lymphatic and urinary system reflexes to eliminate toxic wastes and replace with natural vibrant energy.

Other suggestions

- See Reproductive and Genital Disorders.

HERPES

Genital Herpes

Definition

Inflammatory skin eruptions, in the genital region, with patches of distinct vesicles.

Emotional aspect

Self-punishment or personal rejection due to uneasiness or guilt over having any kind of pleasure, not just sexual.

Reflexes

- As for Reproductive Disorders.
- Concentrate on the central nervous system reflexes, especially the big, fourth and little toes, as well as the middle and lower back reflexes, to release concepts of guilt and self-hatred.
- Circulatory, lymphatic and urinary system reflexes to reduce inflammation and eliminate toxic substances.

Other suggestions

• See Reproductive and Genital Disorders.

Footnote: *Enjoy inner peace and enjoy all pleasurable aspects of life.*

IMPOTENCE

Definition

Reduced or lack of sexual prowess, with erectile dysfunction.

Emotional aspect

Feeling inadequate due to social pressure, guilt or tension.

Reflexes

• As for Reproductive Disorders.
• Concentrate on the central nervous system reflexes, especially the solar plexus reflexes, to place everything into perspective.
• Reproductive organs, male or female, for self-confidence and sexual prowess.

Other suggestions

• See Reproductive Disorders.
• Health Development Club, 123 Westgate Street, Gloucester GL1 3PC.
• Stay calm. This is an extremely common occurrence. Generally a passing phase!
• Massage both feet and the whole body with aromatherapy essential oils: frankincense, jasmine, lemon, lavender, rose, ylang-ylang.
• Over 120 South American herbs have aphrodisiac qualities!
• Natural remedies: damiana, catuba and ginseng.
• Use lubricants to facilitate lovemaking.
• Partners need to reassure and understand, remove pressure, indulge in foreplay and caress the whole body.

- Homoeopathic remedies: Argent. Nit. – to relieve marked anxiety and deep fear; Arnica – for temporary impotence due to trauma or injury; Lycopodium – for prolonged affliction; Sabal Serrulata – for elderly disability.

LEUCORRHEA

Definition

Thick whitish or clear vaginal discharge due to inflammation and congestion of mucosa in vagina or cervix.

Emotional aspect

Feeling the weaker gender and resenting power of the male.

Reflexes

- As for Reproductive Disorders.
- Spend time on the female reproductive organ reflexes, especially vaginal and cervical reflexes, to ease tension, irritation and discomfort.

Other suggestions

- See Gynaecological Disorders.
- Attend to personal hygiene with regular douches and use of bidets.
- Avoid vaginal deodorants.
- Homoeopathic remedies: Alumina – clears thin watery discharge before and after menstruation; Borax – relieves copious clear discharge mid-cycle; Kreosote – for yellow, watery, acidic discharge; Pulsatilla – especially if burning and acrid.

MENOPAUSE DISORDERS

Definition

Disorders related to the otherwise natural and gradual cessation of menstruation around mid-life. Although associated with the female, this natural transition is often approached with a sense of doom by both males and females due to inappropriate social conditioning.

Emotional aspect

The menopause is nature's gift to women! It offers freedom from child-bearing! Social conditioning interferes with this natural occurrence by instilling self-doubt and fear of no longer being desirable or needed. This rejection of the self arises from a deep fear of getting old or losing sexuality.

Reflexes

- As for Reproductive and Gynaecological Disorders.
- Spend time on the female reproductive organs, concentrating on the uterus reflexes, for natural changes to occur in a calm, relaxed environment.
- Liver, circulatory, lymphatic and urinary system reflexes to release conditioned beliefs and wasted emotions.

Other suggestions

- See Reproductive Disorders.
- Women's Health and Reproduction Right Centre, 52 Featherstone Street, London EC1Y 8RT. Tel: 0171-251 6580
- Think positively!
- Enjoy being your own person without fear of pregnancy or interruptions.
- Eat smaller quantities of wholesome, nourishing food.
- Drink plenty of purified fluids, avoiding alcohol, to reduce hot flushes.
- Take evening primrose oil for a natural transition.
- Take pride in your appearance.
- Natural remedies for hot flushes: Dr. Vogel's menopausal formula MNP 415; Gamma Oryzanol.
- Soya flour, red clover and linseed for plant oestrogen.
- Vitamin C plus Bioflavanoid supplements.
- Osteopathy or acupuncture to ease any discomfort.
- Homoeopathic remedies: Caulophyllum – to release nervous tension, emotional instability and excessive anxiety;

Cimicifuga – for irritability, restlessness, depression; Lachesis – useful remedy for menopausal disorders.
- Avoid caffeine, cigarettes, spicy foods, aspirin and other drugs.

Footnote: *Menopause is a time of self-pursuit and actualisation. Go for it!*

MENSTRUAL DISORDERS

Amenorrhoea

Dysmenorrhoea

Definition

Interference, excessive activity or the delayed onset of the natural blood flow from the mucous membrane of the female uterus on a monthly basis.

Amenorrhoea: a lack of blood flow due to pregnancy, anxiety or because too young to menstruate.

Dysmenorrhoea: painful menstruation with dull aches and cramps.

Flooding: excessive blood flow.

Emotional aspect

Confusion, fear, guilt or rejection of female qualities.

Reflexes

- As for Gynaecological Disorders.
- Concentrate on the central nervous system reflexes, particularly the solar plexus reflexes, for loving, creative thoughts to infiltrate mind, body and soul.
- Female reproductive organs to release from the grips of fear and anxiety so that they can function naturally.

Other suggestions

- See Reproductive Disorders.
- Homoeopathic remedies: Baryta Carb – for delayed onset or

of brief duration; Borax – to ease profuse, frequent menstruation; Conium – to regulate irregular periods and ease swollen breasts; Pulsatilla – for severe pain, backache, nausea and palpitations.

Footnote: *Appreciate, with love and understanding, the honour and gift of nurturing newly created life.*

MISCARRIAGE
Abortion

Definition
The spontaneous or assisted premature expulsion and loss of a fetus before it is viable, due to inadequate environmental conditions or the unnatural development of the embryo.

Emotional aspect
Inability to bring in a new soul either due to inappropriate timing or fear about the future.

Reflexes
- As for Reproductive and Gynaecological Disorders.
- Concentrate on the central nervous system reflexes, especially the big, fourth and fifth toes, as well as the solar plexus reflexes, for peace of mind and restoration of faith in the self.
- Female reproductive organs reflexes to release the womb from the grips of fear and disappointment.

Other suggestions
- See Reproductive Disorders.
- Miscarriage Association, c/o Clayton Hospital, Northgate, Wakefield, West Yorkshire WF1 3JS. Tel: 01924 200799
- The Stillbirth and Neonatal Death Society (SANDS), 28 Portland Place, London W1N 4DE. Tel: 0171-436 7940
- Issue – The National Fertility Association, 509 Aldridge Road, Birmingham B44 8NA. Tel: 0121 344 4414

- Support for Termination of Abnormality (SAFTA), 29/30 Soho Square, London W1V 6JB. Tel: 0171-439 6124
- Acknowledge the profound loss and understand your anger, grief and depression. Fully express your emotions.
- Keep physically and psychologically healthy in preparation for any future pregnancies.
- Rest to allow mind, body and soul to readjust.
- Give up smoking and reduce alcohol intake to prepare a satisfactory environment for future pregnancies.
- If Rhesus negative, request an anti D injection, to prevent the production of antigens.
- Homoeopathic remedies: Arnica – to relieve shock, if due to trauma or injury; Chamomilla – if due to excessive nervous excitement; Sabina – for threatened symptoms early in pregnancy.

Footnote: *Everything has its time and place. The more confusing and unjust, the greater the opportunity to understand the self.*

OVARIES

See Endocrine Glands

OVARY DISORDERS

See Endocrine Glands

PREMENSTRUAL SYNDROME (PMS)

Definition

Emotional and physical changes prior to menstruation.

Emotional aspect

Influence from outside forces. Inner turmoil and confusion. Rejecting certain aspects of feminity.

Reflexes

- As for Gynaecological Disorders.
- Spend time on the female reproductive system reflexes for ease with feminity.

Other suggestions

- National Association for Premenstrual Syndrome, P.O. Box 72, Sevenoaks, Kent TN13 1XQ.
- See Menstrual and Reproductive Disorders.

PREGNANCY

PREGNANCY DISORDERS

Definition

The nurturing of a fertilised egg in the womb giving it time to grow and develop sufficiently to survive on its own. Tension interferes with this miraculous development by constricting the blood flow to the womb and depriving the growing fetus of life-forces. It can also cause pain and discomfort in the mother's body.

Morning sickness: the unnatural occurrence of nausea and vomiting.
Back pain: generally in the lower or middle back.
Haemorrhoids: locally dilated rectal veins.
Varicose veins: distended, twisted veins, usually in the legs.
Constipation: incomplete or inactive bowel movements.
Flatulence: excessive gas in stomach or bowels.
Exhaustion: total lack of strength.

These conditions are **not** symptoms of pregnancy. Pregnancy should be the best time of a woman's life!

Emotional aspects

A true gift of life! Unfortunately due to social conditioning, unrealistic expectations and inadequate preparation dis-ease sets in with feelings of insecurity and uncertainty.

Morning sickness: extreme subconscious nervousness.
Wondering whether going to cope or whether will be able to
stomach the impending changes!
Back pain: if lower back, anxiety regarding finances, security
and support. If middle back, feeling concerned and possibly
guilty about actions.
Haemorrhoids: feeling weighed down, overburdened or
anxious about the delivery.
Varicose veins: feeling discouraged and pressurised. Disliking
present circumstances.
Constipation: feeling insecure. Fearful of letting go.
Flatulence: extreme fear gripping the insides.
Exhaustion: wanting to escape momentarily because
everything seems to be getting on top. Not coping.

Reflexes

* For the first three months the embryo is reflected on to the
  inner aspect of **one of the feet**, unless it is a multiple birth, in
  which case it is reflected onto both feet! They vibrate to
  red/orange.

* As the pregnancy develops and the baby grows so too do the
  swellings on the feet as they spread on to the fleshy insteps
  on the heels. It is occasionally possible to detect the baby's
  position, with the smaller swelling being the baby's head and
  the larger swelling the baby's body! They vibrate to
  red/orange/yellow/green.

* Reflexology, sensitively applied, is **excellent** during
  pregnancy! It calms the mother, and creates an ideal
  environment in which the fetus can grow. The baby after the
  birth is consequently more content, vibrant and healthy.

* For individual disorders refer to relevant sections.

* During childbirth, reflexology is invaluable in helping relax
  the mother so that the uterine muscles are nurtured, reducing
  the discomfort, and making space in the birth canal to ease
  the birth of the baby.

- After childbirth, reflexology provides the mother with the strength to cope and enjoy her baby and allows her body to return with ease to its natural state. Since the mother is calm, her milk flows freely and the baby is content. Within a tranquil environment, the baby can grow and develop with ease.

Other suggestions

- Massage both feet with aromatherapy essential oils to further enhance development in peaceful surroundings: camomile, geranium, grapefruit, jasmine, lavender, rose. For digestive upsets – cardamom, coriander, dill; For nausea – above plus fennel, lavender; For cramp – cypress, geranium, lavender; For oedema – cypress, ginger, lavender; After the birth – calendula, clary sage, fennel, frankincense, geranium, neroli.
- During childbirth massage both feet with aromatherapy essential oils for inner peace and the strength to cope. Rose – relaxes uterine muscles; neroli – calms nerves; lavender – stimulates circulation; nutmeg – has analgesic properties; clary sage – assists the birth; geranium – uplifts the spirits!
- Play dolphin and classical music throughout the pregnancy, delivery and postnatally.
- Eat wholesome, natural foods to nurture the whole.
- Drink plenty of purified drinks.
- Relaxation techniques for peace of mind.
- Parenthood classes for both parents.
- Bach flower remedies, especially Rescue Remedy, for the ability to cope.

Footnote: *The gift of life is the greatest gift of all! Treasure it!*

PROSTATE

Definition

A gland deep in the male pelvis, below the bladder, which is associated with the genital organs. It surrounds the male urethra and is a vital part of masculinity and the reproductive process. It secretes seminal fluid through which sperm is transported.

Emotional aspect

Symbolises the masculine principle.

Reflexes

- The prostate reflexes to enhance masculinity.

Other suggestions

- Enjoy regular lovemaking.
- Eat oysters for their high level of zinc for natural functioning!

PROSTATE DISORDERS

Definition

Interference with the functioning of the prostate.
  Prostate hypertrophy: an enlargement of the fibrous and
  glandular tissue which inhibits the flow of urine.

Emotional aspect

Feeling pressurised sexually or anxious thoughts that interfere
with masculinity.

Reflexes

- As for Reproductive Disorders.
- Spend time on the male reproductive organs, particularly the
  prostate reflexes, to boost masculine characteristics.

Other suggestions

- See Reproductive and Prostate Disorders.
- Turn on a tap and run water to encourage urination.

STERILITY

INFERTILITY

Definition

Fertilisation and reproduction are not possible due to barrenness
of either male or female.

Emotional aspect

Possible sub-conscious fear of and/or resistance to becoming a parent. Inhibiting the natural flow and process of life.

Reflexes

- Regular reflexology treatments on both partners create ideal circumstances and a natural environment for fertilisation (provided there is no physical obstruction such as scarred, blocked fallopian tubes) by simply relaxing the whole. See figures 000–000.
- Central nervous system reflexes, particularly the big, fourth and fifth toes, for a productive mind.
- Endocrine system reflexes, especially the pituitary, pineal, testes or ovary gland reflexes, for emotional balance and a stable internal environment.
- Male or female reproductive organ reflexes for natural nurturing abilities.
- Circulatory, lymphatic and urinary system reflexes to release resistance to the cycle of life.
- All bodily reflexes for overall well-being.

Other suggestions

- See Reproductive Disorders.
- Eat wholesome, natural foods to nurture the whole.
- Vitamin and mineral supplements if required.
- Men: wear loose trousers and have tepid baths for the ideal environment and temperature for natural sperm production.
- Avoid excessive alcohol, caffeine, nicotine and fats.
- Eliminate drugs and nicotine intake.
- Lovemaking unites two people with a special bond and should always be a mutually exhilarating act of unconditional love.

SYPHILIS

Definition

Venereal disease from sexual intercourse, or contact with infected matter. There are three stages of development, but with the advancement of medical technology, syphilis rarely progresses beyond the first stage.

Emotional aspect

Letting go of personal strength and values.

Reflexes

- Central nervous system reflexes, concentrating on all reflexes, for a shift in consciousness and to allow the healthy formation of new brain and nerve tissue.
- Endocrine system reflexes, concentrating on all gland reflexes, for emotional control and inner strength.
- Circulatory system reflexes, especially the heart reflexes, for a vibrant flow of natural life-forces.
- Male or female reproductive system reflexes for growth of natural cells.
- Lymphatic and urinary reflexes to eliminate toxic substances.
- Reflexes of affected areas (see foot chart) to encourage the free exchange of essential life-forces and toxic substances.

Other suggestions

- See Reproductive Disorders.
- Avoid contact with others until it has healed.
- Utilise time profitably by pursuing constructive, enjoyable, rewarding activities.
- Unconditionally love the self.

TESTICLES DISORDERS

Testes

See Endocrine System

UTERUS

Definition

Triangular, hollow, muscular womb situated in the pelvis. Part of the female reproductive system that nourishes and guards the developing fetus during pregnancy.

Emotional aspect

Nurtures and protects the creation of life.

Reflexes

- **Uterine reflexes** for total nourishment and protection.

Characteristics

- Swollen reflexes: either overprotection or weighed down by female responsibilities, about to menstruate or indicates pregnancy!
- Flattened reflexes: exhausted with trying to cater to female aspects of life.
- Broken veins over reflexes: perceived emotional or physical abuse of feminity. Harbouring hurt feelings.

Other suggestions

- Massage both feet and body with aromatherapy essential oils to enhance feminity: jasmine, neroli, patchouli, rose, rosewood, sandalwood.
- Relaxation techniques for inner peace.
- To look good is to feel good!
- Bach flower remedies for self-confidence and self-acceptance.

VAGINITIS

Definition

Inflammation of vagina.

Emotional aspect

Anger at females being regarded as the more vulnerable sex.

Reflexes

- As for Reproductive and Vaginal Disorders.
- Spend time on the liver reflexes to release pent-up emotions.
- Female reproductive system reflexes, concentrating on the vaginal reflexes, to eliminate inflamed cells and make space for vibrant, healthy cell formation.

Other suggestions

- See Reproductive Disorders.
- Regular douches.
- Homoeopathic remedies: Calcarea – for milky white discharge; China – if also feeling extremely weak; Platina – relieves watery, itchy discharge. Sepia – for yellowish–green discharge.

Footnote: *Valued aspects of life are protected by cosmic law, so respect and love the female form and others will do the same.*

VENEREAL DISEASE

See also AIDS, Gonorrhoea, Herpes, Syphilis

Definition

Disorders introduced mainly through sexual intercourse.

Emotional aspect

The meaning of the act of lovemaking is lost, abused or disregarded for selfish reasons.

Reflexes

- As for Reproductive Disorders.
- Spend time on the male or female reproductive organs to promote healing.
- Lymphatic and circulatory system reflexes for the free flow of life-forces and to flush through toxic substances.

Other suggestions

- See Reproductive Disorders.

Footnote: *The act of lovemaking unites the energies of two people who care deeply enough for one another to form one creative loving energy.*

URINARY SYSTEM

Definition

Filters excessive fluids and toxic substances from the blood for excretion from the body to keep it free of toxic substances and to maintain a stable internal watery environment.

Emotional aspect

Determine which ideas, emotions and feelings are no longer of value so that they can be filtered out and eliminated.

Reflexes

Kidney reflexes, found immediately below the hollows at the bases of hard balls of both feet, with the **right** kidney reflex being fractionally lower and slightly more towards inner edge of foot. They are massaged for the efficient filtering and secretion of toxic substances and vibrate to orange.

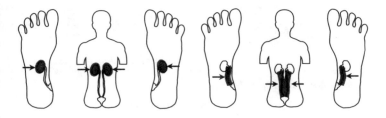

Kidney reflexes   Ureter reflexes

Ureter reflexes run from the centres of the kidney reflexes to the swellings below the ridge of bone, on the inner aspect of both feet, and are massaged to ease the flow of urine from the kidney to the bladder. They vibrate to orange/red.

Bladder reflexes are swellings on the inner aspects of both feet, below the bony ridges, and are massaged for the relaxed expansion and contraction of the reservoir, so that urine can be naturally accommodated and stored until it is ready for expulsion. They vibrate to orange/red.

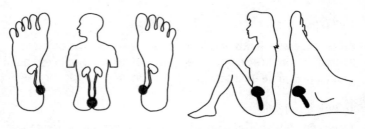

Bladder reflexes   *Bladder & Urethral reflexes*

Female Urethral reflexes run from the bladder reflexes to the hollows midway between the inner ankles and the tips of the heels. They vibrate to red.

Male Urethral reflexes stretch from the bladder reflexes to the tips of the heels and are massaged to strengthen muscular sphincters for the efficient storage and expulsion of urine. They vibrate to red.

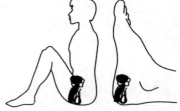

Bladder & Urethral reflexes

Characteristic reflexes

- Swollen kidney reflexes: filled with anxiety and frustration.
- Flattened kidney reflexes: exhausted from trying to sort out wasted emotions.
- Swollen bladder reflexes: holding onto resentment, usually towards a loved one.
- Flattened bladder reflexes: drained of emotion.

Other suggestions

- At birth there is no conscious control of the urethral muscles, but around 18 months to 3 years, the urethral orifices naturally strengthen.

- Drink plenty of purified water, particularly after a reflexology massage, to flush through latent waste products.
- Avoid upsetting the sodium/potassium balance with too high a salt intake. Counteract this by increasing the amount of water taken.

Footnote: *Life is an ongoing cycle – for progression the old needs to give way to the new.*

BLADDER DISORDERS

Definition

Interference with the bladder function due to tension or infection.

Emotional aspect

Difficulty in releasing outdated emotions and limiting belief systems.

Reflexes

- Concentrate on the nervous system, especially the big, fourth and little toes, as well as the midbrain and solar plexus reflexes, to open the mind, release fear and strengthen subconscious control of the bladder sphincters.
- Endocrine system reflexes for inner strength and emotional understanding.
- Urinary system, particularly the bladder reflexes, to free from the grips of tension and to facilitate function.
- Lymphatic system reflexes for the free flow of toxic elimination.

Other suggestions

- Seek professional guidance.
- Massage both feet, concentrating on the toes and instep, with aromatherapy essential oils to release the musculature from the grips of tension: basil, cinnamon, clove, coriander, eucalyptus, fennel, hyssop, lavender, marjoram, pine,

rosemary; to accelerate healing: cajeput, cinnamon, coriander, cumin, clove, fennel, hyssop, oregano, niaouli, pine.
- Bach flower remedies for ease with the self.
- Herbal remedies: asparagus, carrot, parsley, pawpaw.
- Homoeopathic remedy: Nux Vomica – to relieve tearing pain; Opium – to sensitise a 'paralysed' bladder; Camphor – to calm spasms; Causticum – for the retention of urine, especially after an operation.

BRIGHT'S DISEASE

NEPHRITIS

Definition

Inflammation of one or both kidneys from hypersensitivity to toxic substances.

Emotional aspect

Feeling inflamed and extremely angry with the continual disappointments and disillusionments in life. Failing to achieve satisfactory results.

Reflexes

- As for Kidney Disorders.
- Concentrate on the kidney reflexes, to release past disappointments and ease interaction with the environment.

Other suggestions

- See Kidney Disorders.

Footnote: *What lies behind and what lies ahead are insignificant to what lies in the present. If the present is disagreeable, change it! People do not resist change, they resist being changed! Success lies in acknowledging the here and now and making the most of every moment.*

CYSTITIS

Definition

Inflammation of the bladder, and sometimes the urethral outlet, with painful frequent urination. More common in females.

Emotional aspect

Anger and frustration at basic insecurity. Not being able to express and release bursting emotions.

Reflexes

- Central nervous system, especially the big, fourth and fifth toes, as well as the solar plexus reflexes, to ease the extreme pain to allow for free exchange of progressive thoughts.
- Endocrine system reflexes, particularly the pituitary, thymus and adrenal gland reflexes to reduce rigors, fevers and inflamed emotions for inner harmony.
- Liver reflexes to release feelings of anger and frustration.
- Urinary reflexes, concentrating on the bladder and urethral reflexes, to release from the grips of frustration for the free expression of emotions.
- Circulatory and lymphatic system reflexes to assist in the elimination of toxic substances and to allow enhanced distribution of essential life-forces to nurture the whole.

Other suggestions

- See Bladder Disorders.
- Drink plenty of purified fluids.

Footnote: *Create a happier, peaceful reality by allowing everyone, particularly the self, space for unlimited expression.*

ENURESIS

Definition

Involuntary release of urine and inability to control the bladder during sleep. If control of urine is not naturally acquired around 3 years, the condition is considered to be enuresis.

Emotional aspect

Deep-seated fear of being out of control and insecure. During childhood, perceived parental displeasure threatens a child's security.

Reflexes

- See Bladder Disorders.
- The parents, as well as the child, should have regular reflexology massage for the strength and understanding to respond appropriately.
- Spend time on the urinary system reflexes, specifically the bladder and urethral sphincter reflexes, to release from the grips of anxiety so that urine can be naturally retained and expelled.

Other suggestions

- Enuresis Resources and Information Centre (ERIC), 65 St. Michael's Hill, Bristol BS2 8DZ.
- Seek professional guidance.
- Although distressing for all concerned, keep calm and be understanding and supportive at all times.
- Look into the possibility of a temporary emotional upset, for example, a new baby, moving house, death of a loved one, and deal with it.
- Restrict fluid intake after lunch.
- The child should urinate before going to sleep and keep a potty by the bed.
- Have a torch or lamp within easy reach.
- Set an alarm for midnight and for early morning.
- Sleep on the bottom bunk.
- Homoeopathic remedies: Arsenicum – for the overconscientious child; Belladonna – if the wet phases occur during the early hours of the morning; Ferr. Phos. – to strengthen sphincter control and reduce the coffee smell; Gelsemium – to calm the nervous, highly strung child; Sabadilla – for general bladder weakness.

Footnote: *Unconditionally love and accept all concerned.*

INCONTINENCE

Definition

Loss of bladder function with inability to control natural functions and secretions.

Emotional aspect

Unable to hold on to or control emotions that have steadily built up over the years.

Reflexes

- As for Bladder Disorders.
- Spend time on the urinary tract reflexes, especially the bladder and urethral sphincter reflexes, to strengthen the muscles for natural functioning.

Other suggestions

- See Bladder Disorders.
- Seek professional guidance to check that the condition is not due to infection.
- Pelvic floor exercises and relaxation techniques.
- Homoeopathic remedies: Causticum – for constant dribbling and the involuntary release of urine with laughter; Ferrum Phos. – to strengthen control.

KIDNEY DISORDERS

Definition

Interference with the natural process of filtering and eliminating toxic substances causing an imbalance due to tension, infection or obstruction.

Emotional aspect

Feeling a failure. Difficulty in sifting through emotions to release outdated feelings and limiting belief systems.

Reflexes

- Central nervous system reflexes, particularly the big, third and fourth toes, as well as the spinal and solar plexus reflexes, to ease the mind, elevate consciousness and provide support.
- Concentrate on the facial, neck and shoulder reflexes to prevent or relieve swelling and water retention.
- Endocrine system reflexes, especially the pituitary, thymus and adrenal gland reflexes, for inner harmony and emotional strength.
- Digestive system reflexes to ease peristalsis.
- Liver reflexes to eliminate inflamed emotions.
- Ankle reflexes to prevent or relieve swelling and water retention (oedema).
- Concentrate on the kidney reflexes, to release past disappointments and ease interaction within the environment.
- Circulatory and lymphatic system reflexes for the natural distribution of essential life-forces and the elimination of toxic wastes.

Other suggestions

- Seek professional guidance.
- Drink plenty of purified water, particularly after a reflexology massage, to flush through latent waste products.
- Avoid upsetting the sodium/potassium balance with too high a salt intake. Counteract this by increasing the amount of water taken.
- Elevate the feet, especially if swollen.
- Drink plenty of purified fluids.
- Eat wholesome nutrients with reduced protein content, salt and spicy additives.
- Control sodium intake.
- Periodically drink only purified water for a day, to rest the kidneys.
- Relaxation techniques for inner peace.
- Bach flower remedies to release anguish and despair.
- Massage both feet, particularly the toes and insteps, with

aromatherapy essential oils to help reduce inflammation: camomile, clary sage, fennel, lemon, lavender, neroli, rose.

KIDNEY STONES

Definition
Deposits of granular substances within the kidney tubules causing severe renal colic.

Emotional aspect
Collections of unresolved frustration and disillusionment.

Reflexes
- As for Kidney Disorders.
- Concentrate on the urinary system reflexes, to relax the tubules and encourage expulsion of the kidney stones.

Other suggestions
- See Kidney Disorders.

PYELONEPHRITIS

Definition
Inflammation of the pelvic area of the kidney and its contents.

Emotional aspect
Inflamed at the disappointments and frustrations in life.

Reflexes
- As for Kidney Disorders.
- Spend time on the liver reflexes to release inflamed emotions.
- Urinary system reflexes to flush through hampering emotions.

Other suggestions
- See Kidney Disorders.

URINARY INFECTIONS

Definition

Inflammation of the urinary tract.

Emotional aspect

Anger at the build-up of emotional hurts and frustrations.

Reflexes

- As for Bladder and Kidney Disorders.
- Concentrate on the liver reflexes to release pent-up emotions and urinary system reflexes to accelerate the healing process.

Other suggestions

- See Bladder and Kidney Disorders.
- Wholesome, natural foods, excluding salt and spices.
- Drink plenty of purified fluids.

Footnote: *Lovingly release past emotions, realising that each life has its own pattern for the purpose of personal development and growth.*

SKIN

Definition
Outer protective, flexible continuous covering of the body. A sensitive organ.

Emotional aspect
Senses environmental changes and protects unique characteristics of the individual.

Reflexes
- All reflexes on both feet.

Other suggestions
- Care for the skin by keeping it clean, supple and healthy.
- Enjoy wholesome, natural foods to nurture new cells.
- Drink plenty of purified fluids to keep whole system fresh.
- Have regular herbal and aroma facials.

SKIN DISORDERS

Definition
Overreaction resulting in extreme irritability or tension causing physical blemishes.

Emotional aspect
Burying and storing past fears and anxieties that threaten personal security. Oversensitivity. Emotions surface causing irritability and possibly erupting. Situations or people 'getting under the skin'.

Reflexes
The nature and colouring of the skin on the feet continually changes as subconscious thoughts and moods swing. Many

different colourings can be detected at any one time. The position of the colouring is significant.

Flesh coloured: balanced and healthy.

White: drained, exhausted, washed out.

Red: angry or embarrassed.

Yellow: very disillusioned.

Green: envious.

Blue/black: deep emotional hurts.

Flaking skin: extreme irritability.

Shiny skin: emotional friction, and continually rubbing up against resistance.

Transparent skin: vulnerability.

Hard skin: protection against the outside or concealing and protecting true emotions.

Cracked skin: feeling divided.

- As for Skin Disorders.
- Central nervous system reflexes, especially the brain and solar plexus reflexes, to increase the level of tolerance and calm irritable nerves.
- Concentrate on the eye reflexes to desensitise.
- Endocrine system reflexes, particularly the pituitary, pineal, thymus and adrenal gland reflexes for emotional control and to build up defence mechanisms.
- Shoulder reflexes to take the 'weight off the shoulders'.
- Liver reflexes to relieve built-up irritability.
- Lymphatic reflexes to flush through irritants and increase immunity.
- Reflexes of the affected areas for overall tranquillity.

Other suggestions

- If severe, seek professional guidance.
- Massage both feet, especially the toes, with aromatherapy essential oils for deeper inner peace and greater understanding: camomile, fennel, lavender, lemon, tagetes, yarrow; for infection: tea tree; to invigorate: camomile, carrot, cyprus, eucalyptus, fennel, geranium, rose.
- Soothe irritated area with lavender aromatherapy oil.

- Use cotton sheets and wear natural fibres.
- Eat wholesome, natural foods avoiding colourants, preservatives and additives.
- Drink plenty of purified fluids.
- Relaxation techniques for inner tranquillity.
- Bach flower remedies to calm the mind.
- Homoeopathic remedies: Agaricus – for chilblains and red, painful, itchy, cracked skin; Natrum Mur – to ease cracks around the nails; Petroleum – to relieve thick, dirty eczema; Silicea – for deep cracks that fail to heal.

Footnote: *Experience freedom by releasing the mind.*

ALLERGIES

Definition

Acute hypersensitivity of skin and conjunctiva of eyes.

Emotional aspect

Others are perceived and seen to be irritating and getting under the skin.

Reflexes

- As for Skin Disorders.

Other suggestions

- As for Skin Disorders.

ABSCESS

Definition

Collection of pus in a cavity beneath the skin.

Emotional aspect

Accumulation of suppressed emotional hurts that have festered, but by seeking an outlet come to the surface and erupt.

Reflexes

- As for Skin Disorders.
- The abscess may initially get worse because it needs to form a head to release the pus.
- Concentrate on the specific reflex for the affected area for the natural eruption and discharge.

Other suggestions

- See Skin Disorders.

ACNE

Definition

Chronic inflammation of the skin's sebaceous ducts. Hard, painful eruptions occur mainly on the face, neck, chest and back.

Emotional aspect

Frustration and anger at difficulty in controlling and dealing with life's natural transitions, for example, from childhood to adulthood or from one phase of life to another.

Reflexes

- As for Skin Disorders.
- Concentrate on the specific reflexes of the affected areas:
  Scalp reflexes to clear irritable thoughts and dandruff.
  Face reflexes for the courage to face the world.
  Neck reflexes for free expression and acceptance of the true self.
  Back and shoulder reflexes for inner strength and the ability to cope.
- All bodily reflexes for overall enthusiasm.

Other suggestions

- See Skin Disorders.
- Enjoy creative, rewarding activities to boost self-esteem.

- Tea-tree aromatherapy essential oil directly on the spot to reduce inflammation and promote healing.
- Homoeopathic remedies: Kali. Brom. – to relieve acne on face, neck and upper back; Sulphur – to ease infected, painful eruptions; Psorinum – for severe infection; Kali. Sulph. – to pacify oversensitive skin.
- Acne on face and neck: regular herbal and cleansing facials.

Footnote: *Avoid comparisons with others and allow individual talents to colour the world with imagination and ingenuity.*

ATHLETE'S FOOT

Definition
Fungal infection with flaking skin between toes.

Emotional aspect
Extreme irritability that gets under the skin. Others constantly interfere, doubt and question ideas, thereby hindering progress.

Reflexes
Due to its contagious nature, the afflicted person should massage his/her *own feet*. Initially, others should avoid physical contact with the affected areas, although the auric space can be massaged. Afterwards, wash your hands thoroughly with a disinfectant to avoid the possible risk of spreading infection.

- As for Skin Disorders.
- Concentrate on the sinus reflexes to reduce irritability, eye reflexes for a clearer outlook and ear reflexes to open the ears to other opinions.
- All reflexes on both feet for a firm foundation from which to step ahead with joy and confidence.

Other suggestions
- See Skin Disorders.
- Apply aromatherapy essential oils directly to the affected area with cotton wool, to accelerate healing: lavender, lemon, tea-tree.

BLISTERS

SHINY SKIN

Definition

A blister is a vesicle filled with serum and shiny skin is smoothness on the skin's surface. Both are caused from friction of consistently rubbing up against resistance.

Emotional aspect

Constant emotional friction. Rubbing up against other ideas and belief systems.

Reflexes

- For a blister on the foot, gently rest thumb or finger on or over the afflicted area and allow the free exchange of energy to pulsate through.
  The position of the blister and shiny skin on the feet indicates specific areas of emotional friction:
  Toes: conflict of thoughts and intellect.
  Necks: worn out from expressing or swallowing conflicting ideas.
  Balls: friction within the environment or with feelings of self-worth or matters concerning the heart.
  Upper instep: constant resistance and friction regarding activities.
  Lower instep: friction within relationships or resistance when communicating.
  Heels: continual obstructions and friction inhibiting development, progress and mobility.

Other suggestions

- Place neat camomile or lavender aromatherapy essential oils directly on to the blister.

Footnote: *Go with the flow!*

BOIL (FURUNCLE)

CARBUNCLE

Definition

A boil is a suppurative, painful swelling due to acute inflammation of the skin and subcutaneous tissue around the hair. A hard and round swelling with a central core of dead tissue. Eventually it is discharged or re-absorbed. A carbuncle is similar to a collection of boils.

Emotional aspect

Unexpressed fury at others or situations for getting under the skin.

Reflexes

- As for Skin Disorders.
- Spend time on the affected site reflexes to ease the pain and increase the supply of essential nutrients for healing.

Other suggestions

- Apply poultices twice a day to the area: crushed nasturtium seeds wrapped in a bandage and wrung out with hot water.
- Bach flower remedies to cleanse the whole.
- Homoeopathic remedies: Hepar Sulph – to mature the boil; Hypericum Tincture – apply to the boil to ease extreme sensitivity and pain; Tarentula – for extremely acute, throbbing pain.

BRUISING

Definition

Superficial injury to the skin rupturing the blood vessels which bleed into the subcutaneous tissue.

Emotional aspect

Emotional knocks of the self arising from extreme sensitivity.

Reflexes

- As for Skin Disorders.
- Concentrate on the central nervous system reflexes, especially the solar plexus reflexes, to ease the pain and reduce sensitivity.
- Reflexes of the affected areas (see foot chart) to reduce swelling, discoloration, sensitivity and to promote healing.

Other suggestions

- See Skin Disorders.
- Cold compress to reduce the reaction and ease pain.
- Massage the affected area with aromatherapy essential oils to assist with the absorption of blood from the subcutaneous tissue: geranium, hyssop, lavender.
- Arnica homoeopathic oil, cream, ointment, gel and tablets.

Footnote: *Feel at ease with the self and those within the vicinity.*

BURNS

Definition

Injury to the skin and subcutaneous tissue from radiation or direct external heat.

Emotional aspect

Consuming anger that erupts from within, especially when feelings of insecurity are present.

Reflexes

- As for Skin Disorders.
- Rest the third finger lightly on or just above the burn reflexes on the feet to allow free exchange of energy to promote healing.
- Spend time on the liver reflexes to release consuming anger.
- Reflexes of affected area to relieve pain, congestion, swelling, discomfort and redness.

Other suggestions
- See Skin Disorders.
- Apply ice-cold water, ice, neat lavender or butter immediately to the burned area.
- Homoeopathic remedies: Arnica – for shock; Cantharis – to ease burning pain; Hypericum – apply locally, except in severe cases; Sulphur – for mild scalds and minor burns; Urtica – for marked swelling of less severe burns.

Footnote: *Look within for inner peace and tranquillity and allow it to radiate outwardly for the benefit of all.*

CALLOUSES

Definition
Physical hardening of the skin to protect a specific bodily part.

Emotional aspect
Callous means 'unfeeling' or 'insensitive'. Hard skin builds up, especially on the feet, to protect a specific reflex emotionally and shield the self from callous attack. It may also arise from extreme insecurity, determination, obstinacy or an attempt to conceal the truth. The position of the callous on the feet is significant.

Toe pads: protects or conceals true thought processes and ideas.

Necks of toes: protection or concealment of honest exchange of expression.

Hard ball: protects or conceals heartfelt feelings and own identity.

Instep: protection or concealment of open activity or honest communication.

Heels: protects or conceals security, sexuality, direction or movements. Also from 'digging in the heels!'

Reflexes
- As for Skin Disorders.
- Concentrate on the affected areas to calm and reassure.

Other suggestions

- Massage both feet and the callous with aromatherapy essential oils: carrot, tagetes.
- Regular pedicures and chiropody treatments to remove excessive skin layers.
- Soak the feet in a foot bath with lavender or fennel.
- Although footwear is not the cause, it can aggravate.
- Walk barefoot whenever possible.

CARBUNCLE

See Boils

COLD SORE

Definition

Eruption of festering skin around the mouth, commonly due to the herpes virus.

Emotional aspect

Fuming at the mouth from having to seal the lips and conceal angry words of condemnation.

Reflexes

- As for Skin Disorders.
- Concentrate on the facial reflexes, especially the mouth reflexes, to enhance the healing process.
- Neck, throat and shoulder reflexes to open channels of communication.

Other suggestions

- Add a combination of the following aromatherapy essential oils to a lip gloss base and apply daily: camomile, geranium, lavender, lemon, tea-tree.

Footnote: *Verbally and openly express joyful, loving thoughts.*

CORNS

Definition

Local hardening and thickening of the skin, usually on the toes, to provide physical protection.

Emotional aspect

Protecting ideas from being trampled upon. Reluctance to release past emotional trauma.

Reflexes

- As for Skin Disorders.
- Rest the third finger lightly against the corns on the feet for a free exchange of energy.
- Central nervous system, particularly the solar plexus reflexes, for belief in the self and own ideas.
- Endocrine system reflexes for emotional security and inner understanding.
- Spend time on the liver reflexes to release past emotions.
- Feet reflexes to speed the healing process.

Other suggestions

- See Skin Disorders.

Footnote: *Free the self and think clearly to realise full potential.*

ECZEMA

See also Allergies

Definition

Variety of inflamed skin eruptions with redness, irritation and multiple small vesicles, serous discharge and crusting. Occasional constitutional disturbances. Believed to be a reaction to an allergen or irritant. Associated with asthma and hay fever.

Emotional aspect

Suppressed irritability at others getting under the skin. Emotions fester beneath the skin's surface and erupt at times of extreme anxiety or during periods of total relaxation.

Reflexes

- Concentrate on the central nervous system, especially the spinal and solar plexus reflexes, to reduce anxiety and irritability.
- Endocrine system reflexes, particularly the pituitary, pineal, thymus and adrenal gland reflexes, to stimulate steroid secretion and reduce inflammation. Also for emotional control.
- Concentrate on the reflexes of the affected areas to release from the grips of fearful insecurity and to allow healing to occur.
- Liver reflexes to eliminate festering emotions.
- Circulatory, lymphatic and urinary system reflexes to enhance the distribution of essential life-forces and to release toxic substances.
- All bodily reflexes to ease overall discomfort and for inner tranquillity.

Other suggestions

- See Skin Disorders.
- National Eczema Society, 163 Eversholt Street, London NW1 1BU.
- Massage the affected reflexes, with aromatherapy essential oils to ease irritability: camomile, tagetes, yarrow.
- Use aqueous cream rather than soap to wash.
- Homoeopathic remedies: Graphites – for scalp eruptions; Psorinum – to ease very irritable eczema with a grey, greasy, dirty appearance; Rhus Tox – for red, itchy eczema on the hands and wrists; Sulphur – to prevent the scratching of the rough irritable skin.

Footnote: *Control and peace comes from within creating harmony and joy for the self and others.*

FISTULA

Definition

An unnatural passage that connects the cavity of one organ to another, or a cavity to the skin's surface.

Emotional aspect

A temporary obstruction due to deep anxiety and fear. Gripping on to old ideas or emotions which creates physical need for a new outlet.

Reflexes

- As for Skin Disorders.
- Concentrate on the central nervous system reflexes, particularly the brain and solar plexus reflexes, to ease mental torture, release physical and emotional obstructions.
- Reflexes of the affected areas for uniformity of mind, body and soul.

Other suggestions

- See Skin Disorders.

Footnote: *The natural cycles of life provide exciting new dimensions to life.*

FURUNCLE

See Boils

GANGRENE

Definition

Death of tissue due to the deprivation of essential life-forces.

Emotional aspect

Tense destructive thoughts stagnate mental agility, eventually strangulating love and joy from life.

Reflexes

- As for Skin Disorders.
- Concentrate on the circulatory system reflexes, especially the heart reflexes to improve the flow of life-forces so that all cells are nurtured.
- Reflex of specific area(s) to release from the grips of strangulation and to allow the healthy, new tissue to develop.

Other suggestions

- See Skin Disorders.

Footnote: *Like attracts like, so unconditional self-acceptance attracts the unconditional acceptance of others.*

HERPES SIMPLEX

Labial herpes/cold sores

Definition

Inflammatory skin eruptions on the lips or labia.

Emotional aspect

Inflamed eruptions.
  Lips: eruption of bitter words that have been simmering beneath the surface and have not been vocalised.
  Labia: desire for revenge, especially towards the sexual partner.

Reflexes

- As for Skin and Genital Disorders.
- Concentrate on the endocrine system reflexes, especially the pituitary and adrenal gland reflexes to reduce inflammation.
- For cold sores, the facial reflexes particularly the lip, jaw and shoulder reflexes to release from the grips of tension.
- For labial herpes, the female reproductive reflexes, concentrating on the vaginal reflexes, to release tightness and allow healing to occur.

Other suggestions
- See Skin and Genital Disorders.
- Apply geranium directly to the sores.

HIVES

URTICARIA

NETTLE RASH

Definition
Recurrent eruptions of weals, with pale oedematous centres and red margins on the skin, due to hypersensitivity resulting in extreme irritability.

Emotional aspect
Over-sensitivity causing overreaction due to excessive irritation with life and people.

Reflexes
- As for Skin Disorders.
- Concentrate on the affected areas, to reduce skin irritability and make space for healing.

Other suggestions
- See Skin Disorders.
- Add two drops of camomile German with $\frac{1}{4}$ cup of baking powder to bath water.
- Homoeopathic remedies: Aconite – for severe, acute allergic reaction; Sulphur – to ease chronic swelling and itching; Urtica urens – reliable basic remedy.

Footnote: *Create inner peace and tranquillity.*

ITCHING

See Pruritis

Definition

Irritation of the skin.

Emotional aspect

Irritating aspects of life get under the skin causing irritability and restlessness. Itching to move on or to escape uncomfortable or unsatisfactory circumstances.

Reflexes

- As for Skin Disorders.
- Concentrate on the affected areas, for equilibrium.

Other suggestions

- See Skin Disorders.

LUPUS ERYTHEMATOSUS

Definition

The progressive eruption of red scaling patches with round plaque-like weals and characteristic horny layers of skin. Generally on the face causing fine scarring, but if it spreads over the whole body it is known as disseminated lupus erythematosus. Believed to be an auto-immune reaction to sunlight, infection or other unknown causes.

Emotional aspect

Hopelessness at the futility of having to defend the self. Defeatism because life seems so meaningless.

Reflexes

- As for Skin Disorders.
- Concentrate on the central nervous system reflexes to overcome self-inflicted limitations and accept own worth.
- Facial and shoulder reflexes to face the world with confidence.
- All bodily reflexes on both feet to build up overall immunity, reduce vulnerability and promote well-being.

Other suggestions

- See Skin Disorders.

Footnote: *'Worse' times are lesser degrees of the 'best' times of life and, therefore, provide greater scope for growth and development.*

PIMPLES

Definition

Minute papules or pustules.

Emotional aspect

Small angers surfacing.

Reflexes

- As for Skin Disorders.
- Liver reflexes for the natural release of anger.
- Concentrate on the circulatory, lymphatic and urinary system reflexes for the free distribution of essential life-forces and the efficient elimination of toxic substances.

Other suggestions

- See Skin Disorders.
- Steam the face with boiling water with one drop each of bergamot and cypress.
- Regular facials for deep-cleansing of the skin.

Footnote: *Feel at ease with the self and enjoy life to the full.*

PRURITIS

Definition

Extreme irritation of the whole or specific parts of the skin, for example, pruritis ani (irritability of anus).

Emotional aspect

Itching to move away from a situation that gets under the skin. The position of the irritability on the body is relevant:

Anal, pelvic area, feet or hands: itching to move on or away from something or someone who threatens the individual's security.

Lower abdomen, ankles and wrists: longing for peace with something or someone who threatens the pleasures in life.

Upper abdomen, lower arms and legs: need to do something to regain self-control.

Chest, knees and elbows: wanting to feel better about the loving aspects of life.

Shoulders, upper legs and arms: yearning to express the self.

Head: needing to clarify thoughts, ideas and perceptions.

Reflexes

- As for Skin Disorders.
- Spend time on the specific reflexes of the affected areas for free flow of energy and to accelerate the healing process.

Other suggestions

- See Skin Disorders.
- Massage the affected area with aromatherapy essential oils to reduce irritability: nutmeg, pettigraine, sandalwood.

PSORIASIS

Definition

Chronic skin condition with dry, scaly, red, flaky areas without vesicle formation. Generally on knees and elbows and in hairy areas such as the hair itself and armpits, although can be widespread. Not infectious and of unknown origin.

Emotional aspect

Putting up resistance to acknowledging built-up emotion that has been suppressed to protect the self from being hurt. Often triggered off by a traumatic emotional experience.

Reflexes

- As for Skin Disorders.
- Concentrate on the circulatory, lymphatic and urinary system reflexes for conscious or subconscious acknowledgement and the release of past trauma.
- Specific reflexes of affected areas (see foot chart) to enhance healing.

Other suggestions

- See Skin Disorders.
- Relaxation techniques to prevent the condition flaring up with distress.
- Reduce alcohol intake so that the situation is not aggravated.
- Frequent shampoos to remove scalp scabs.
- Use soothing lotion, such as calamine.
- Wear natural fibre clothing to hide the affected areas.
- Homoeopathic remedies: Arsenicum – to relieve burning irritability of thickened skin; Petroleum – for chronic cases with deep fissures; Psorinum – to ease irritability, bleeding and scaling; Sulphur – one of the best remedies.

Footnote: *Within is the capacity to deal with any and every situation.*

RASH

Definition

Superficial eruption of skin in spots or patches.

Emotional aspect

Usually hasty, impetuous, energetic, reckless people who feel frustrated and irritated by the tardiness or disinterest of others.

Reflexes

- As for Skin Disorders.
- Concentrate on the lymphatic system reflexes to flush through toxic substances.

- All bodily reflexes (see foot chart) for inner strength and understanding.

Other suggestions

- See Skin Disorders.

RINGWORM

See Worms (Digestive System)

SAGGING LINES

Wrinkles

Definition

Lack of elasticity causing drooping and marks on the skin.

Emotional aspect

Inability to cope with the emotional weight and pressure due to a perceived lack of support.

Reflexes

- As for Skin Disorders.
- Concentrate on the facial, chin, neck and shoulder reflexes to relax the musculature so that fresh cells can replace those restricted by tension.
- Concentrate on the lymphatic system reflexes to remove unnecessary weight from the whole.

Other suggestions

- See Skin Disorders.
- Apply directly to the skin, mixed in an oil base: fennel – to firm the skin and gives it a youthful appearance; geranium – to rejuvenate the skin; camomile, neroli, rose – to encourage cellular regeneration.
- Avoid alcohol, cigarettes, coffee, tea, sweets, red meats as these tend to clog the pores.
- Consider a herbal facelift!

SCABIES

Definition

Extreme irritability from female itch-mite egg deposits at
intervals in burrows beneath the skin, especially between
creases of the fingers, axillae and groin.

Emotional aspect

Extreme resentment and irritability at others getting under the
skin and perceivably infecting personal thoughts.

Reflexes

- As for Skin Disorders.
- Concentrate on the reflexes of the affected areas (see the foot
  chart) to increase the blood flow for healing and to eliminate
  irritable substances.
- All bodily reflexes (see foot chart) for inner peace.

Other suggestions

- See Skin Disorders.

SCLERODERMA

Definition

Progressive hardening and rigidity of the skin either in patches or
diffusely.

Emotional aspect

Extra protection due to fear of not coping or caring for the self.

Reflexes

- See Skin Disorders.

Other suggestions

- See Skin Disorders.

Footnote: *Allow universal understanding to provide nourishment
and unconditional love.*

ULCERS

Definition

An Erosion or interruption on the surface of the skin or the mucous membrane, often with a pus secretion. Leg ulceration is generally over varicose veins due to poor circulation.

Emotional aspect

Eating away at the self due to feelings of inadequacy or a gripping fear.

Reflexes

- As for Skin Disorders.
- Concentrate on the reflexes of the affected areas (see foot chart) to promote the healing process.

Other suggestions

- See Skin Disorders.
- Rest the affected part and expose as often as possible to accelerate healing.

URTICARIA

See Hives

VERRUCA

PLANTAR WART

Definition

Excessive thickening of the dermis layer causing a small elevation of skin on the soles of the feet. A type of verruca that starts as a small pimple head and grows thick, hard and painful.

Emotional aspect

Extreme frustration and anger at the base and foundation of life. Spreading discontent about future events.

Reflexes

- As for Skin Disorders.
- Spend time on the foot reflexes for a firm foundation.

Other suggestions

- Seek professional guidance. Can be removed with liquid nitrogen or expertly cut out.
- Apply one of the following directly to the wart: dandelion sap; garlic rubbed in lemon juice, castor oil and celandine juice; tea-tree cream or oil; Thuja occidentalis ointment.

VITILIGO

Definition

The absence of skin pigment resulting in white patches.

Emotional aspect

Feeling an outsider and separate from others because of being different.

Reflexes

- As for Skin Disorders.
- Spend time on the circulatory, lymphatic and urinary system reflexes for the free flow of life-forces and to flush through toxic substances.
- All bodily reflexes (see foot chart) for overall well-being.

Other suggestions

- See Skin Disorders.

WARTS

Definition

Rough, horny cauliflower-shaped projections mainly on the knees and knuckles. The body's defence and immune system eventually destroys them.

Emotional aspect

Subconscious projections of intense dislike, fears and repulsiveness.

Reflexes

- As for Skin Disorders.
- Concentrate on the liver reflexes to release intense emotions.
- Reflexes of the affected areas (see foot chart) to replenish energy supply for enhanced healing.

Other suggestions

- See Skin Disorders.
- Seek professional guidance. Caustics may be used to remove the outer layer and destroy structure, or liquid nitrogen to freeze them off.
- Local applications directly to the wart: celandine juice; dandelion sap; tea-tree essential oil; garlic.
- Children love to kiss their warts to the moon and make a wish for them to vanish!

WHITEHEADS

MILIA

Definition

Impacted sebaceous secretions trapped within the porous ducts causing hard, white lumps on the skin.

Emotional aspect

Hanging on to perceptions of distasteful self-image.

Reflexes

- As for Skin Disorders and Pimples.

Other suggestions

- See Skin Disorders.

$\mathcal{G}$ENERAL

ACHES

Definition

Periods of prolonged discomfort.

Emotional aspect

Desire to be in total control due to temporary insecurity.
Resistance to the natural flow of life.

Reflexes

- Central nervous system reflexes, particularly the solar plexus reflexes, to calm the nerves and ease discomfort.
- All endocrine system reflexes for emotional balance and inner security.
- Specific reflex(es) for affected area(s), as well as the neck and shoulder reflexes, to relax the musculature from the grips of tension.
- Liver, circulatory, lymphatic and urinary system reflexes to lighten the load.

Other suggestions

- Breathe into the ache with long, deep breaths.
- Massage the aching part and the feet with aromatherapy essential oils: lavender, lemon, peppermint, rosemary.
- Create time and space for the self.
- Bach flower remedies to ease the soul.
- Relaxation techniques for peace of mind.

ADDICTIONS

Definition

Habitual craving and excessive intake of a substance, such as food, drugs, alcohol or nicotine, beyond the wilful control of the person.

Emotional aspect

Habitual escapism from extreme discontent of the self.

Reflexes

- Concentrate on all central nervous system reflexes, as well as the big toe, to alter the concept of self and reduce dependency.
- Endocrine system reflexes, especially the pituitary, pineal and adrenal gland reflexes, for self-control and self-esteem.
- Eye reflexes to see the truth and see the self in a better light.
- Liver reflexes to purify and energise the whole.
- Digestive reflexes to naturalise functioning and for the full utilisation of nutrients.
- Circulatory, lymphatic and urinary system reflexes to expel toxic substances and circulate new, vibrant feelings of self-acceptance.
- All reflexes for overall strength and well-being.

Other suggestions

- Seek professional guidance.
- Join a local self-help group.
- Massage both feet, especially the toes and instep, with aromatherapy essential oils for inner tranquillity: bergamot, fennel, geranium, grapefruit, lavender, rosemary; to reduce dependency: calendula, camomile, frankincense, lavender, rose.
- Keep busy with an enjoyable creative activity to boost self-esteem.
- Rebirthing and meditation to understand the true self.
- Acupuncture, hypnotherapy, shiatsu.
- Small appetising meals with wholesome, natural foods.
- Vitamin and mineral supplements, particularly vitamins B complex and C.
- Plenty of purified fluids, particularly fruit juices, to cleanse the system.
- Escape to the country to relax and re-establish contact with nature.

ALCOHOLISM

Definition

Addiction to effects of alcohol, leading to excessive, uncontrolled intake with possible appetite loss, vitamin deficiency, peripheral neuritis, visual impairment, cirrhosis of the liver and a progressive personality deterioration.

Emotional aspect

Anger at not acknowledging and confronting truths about the self.

Reflexes

• As for Addictions

Other suggestions

• See Addictions.
• Contact the district health visitor and social worker.
• Join a local Alcoholics Anonymous self-help group.
• Homoeopathic remedy: Nux Vomica – to relieve depression and irritability.
• Take pride in personal appearance.

Footnote: *Nothing is 'good' or 'bad', it is all a matter of perception.*

ALLERGIES

Definition

Hypersensitivity to a foreign substance which, even in small doses, produces a violent physical reaction.

Emotional aspect

Extreme sensitivity to life, a person or a situation. Atmospheric particles, such as pollen, animal hair, etc, physically manifest irritating emotions that have 'got under the skin'. Conditioned belief systems, reinforced through association, trigger off recurrent attacks.

Reflexes

- See Skin Disorders.
- Concentrate on the central nervous system reflexes, especially the solar plexus reflexes, to reduce hypersensitivity and calm the nerves.

Other suggestions

- See Skin Disorders.
- Massage both feet with aromatherapy essential oils to further ease the irritability: Eczema – camomile, frankincense, yarrow; Bee stings – camomile, lavender; Migraine – grapefruit, lavender, peppermint, rosemary.
- Enjoy wholesome, natural foods avoiding all synthetic products, colourants and preservatives.
- Drink plenty of purified or natural water and rooibos tea.

Footnote: *Irritants are perceptions of threat that are as menacing as the imagination allows them to be!*

BAD BREATH

Halitosis

Definition

Unnatural, offensive and foul-smelling breath.

Emotional aspect

Festering emotions. Frustration at having to mull over foul, angry, revengeful thoughts. Swallowing unexpressed distasteful words.

Reflexes

- Central nervous system, especially the solar plexus reflexes, to clear the mind of festering thoughts and shift levels of consciousness.
- Concentrate on the face, mouth and throat reflexes to relax the jaw muscles and to encourage a fresh supply of blood and nutrients.

- Endocrine system reflexes to calm emotions.
- Neck and shoulder reflexes for the free exchange of vibrant, fresh energies.
- Liver reflexes to release accumulated anger.
- All reflexes on both feet for inner harmony and balance.

Other suggestions

- Massage both feet, particularly the toes, with aromatherapy essential oils for inner peace and tranquillity: lavender, lemon, peppermint, tea-tree, thyme. Also use as mouthwash.
- Bach flower remedies for restored faith and self-forgiveness.
- Fennel herb tea.
- Relaxation techniques for the natural release of destructive emotions.
- Homoeopathic remedies: Nux vomica – to release irritability; Pulsatilla – to restore balance; Mercurius – for overall body freshness.
- Suck mints.

BODY ODOUR

Definition

The offensive smell of sweat and perspiration emitted from the body.

Emotional aspect

Self-protective mechanism in emotionally threatening situations. Extreme fear, anxiety and uncertainty. Means of releasing wasted, fearful emotions. 'Smelly' feet indicate a return to basic roots to work through early stages of development. Wild animals are frightened by bodily odours and attack in self-defence.

Reflexes

- Central nervous system, especially the solar plexus reflexes, to calm the nerves and release anxiety.
- Endocrine system, particularly the pituitary, pineal and adrenal reflexes, for inner strength and emotional harmony.

- Lymphatic and urinary system reflexes for the natural elimination of toxic substances.

Other suggestions

- Relaxation techniques for inner peace.
- Massage feet with aromatherapy essential oils to refresh the whole: bergamot, camomile, clary sage, frankincense.
- Personal hygiene, particularly of the offensive areas.
- Bach flower remedies, particularly Rescue Remedy during emergencies for reassurance and inner confidence.
- Homoeopathic remedies: Nux Vomica – to reduce profuse sweating; Silicea – to relieve offensive smelling feet; Mercurius – for unpleasant, fetid perspiration.

CANDIDA ALBICANS

Definition

Yeast cells naturally live on dead tissues. During health they are kept in check by the immunological system. With candida albicans the yeast cells invade the body and create havoc throughout.

Emotional aspect

Anger, frustration and disillusionment at the perceived lack of direction and insecurity of life.

Reflexes

- Concentrate on all central nervous system reflexes, especially the brain and solar plexus reflexes, to alert the mind preventing or improving memory lapses, poor concentration and depression.
- Endocrine system reflexes, particularly the pituitary, pineal, thymus and adrenal gland reflexes to reduce vulnerability and increase inner strength.
- Neck and shoulder reflexes to ease self-expression.
- Reflexes of the affected area to accelerate healing process.

- Respiratory system reflexes for the full expansion of the breath.
- Digestive system reflexes to calm peristaltic activity and to ease any irritability, bloating, flatulence or cramping.
- Liver reflexes for the subconscious release of anger and frustration.
- Circulatory and lymphatic system reflexes to enhance the distribution of the essential life-forces and elimination of toxic substances.
- All bodily reflexes for harmony and peace throughout.

Other suggestions

- Seek professional guidance.
- Massage both feet, particularly the toes, thymus and affected reflexes, with aromatherapy essential oils, to speed healing process and energise the whole: camomile, cajeput, eucalyptus, geranium, lavender, patchouli, rosemary, tea-tree.
- Eat wholesome, natural foods avoiding substances such as sugar, alcohol, carbohydrates, chocolates and pasta on which yeast usually thrives.
- Boost the immunity with vitamin and mineral supplements.
- Relaxation techniques for inner understanding and for trust in the natural flow of life.
- For vaginal thrush wash out with natural yoghurt mixed with geranium, marjoram and patchouli.
- Bach flower remedies for release from the vexations of life.

CANCER

Carcinoma

Definition

A collection of malformed tissue. Tension deprives certain bodily tissues of essential life-forces and space. Natural growth and effective functioning is inhibited and malformation occurs. Toxic build-up compounds the situation.

Emotional aspect

Fear, anger and frustration simmer beneath the surface causing pockets of tension which increase anxiety. These emotions block the way for personal progress and natural growth.

Reflexes

The reflexology massage reverses this unnatural process. Complete relaxation during the alpha state of consciousness can create space and an ideal environment for new cells to grow, develop and function naturally. Meanwhile the malformed cells are absorbed by the lymphatic vessels and are eliminated from the body.

- Concentrate on all the central nervous system reflexes, especially the brain and solar plexus reflexes, to calm the nerves, ease discomfort and open the mind.
- Endocrine system reflexes, particularly the pituitary, pineal, thyroid, thymus and adrenal gland reflexes for emotional harmony, strength and understanding.
- Reflexes of the affected area to release from the grips of tension and to create space for healing.
- Liver reflexes to release unexpressed emotions.
- Circulatory, lymphatic and urinary system reflexes for the natural release of malformed cells and to make space for the free exchange of essential life-forces to nourish new, healthy cells.
- All bodily reflexes to revitalise and energise the whole.

Other suggestions

- Seek professional guidance.
- Contact the local authority, health visitor and social worker.
- Cancer Help Centre, Grove House, Cornwallis Grove, Clifton, Bristol BS8 4PG.
- Oxygen or ozone therapy to accelerate destruction of the malformed cells.
- Massage both feet with aromatherapy essential oils: clary sage, fennel, geranium, lavender, rose.
- Inspirational books and tapes on attitudinal healing.

- Relaxation techniques to create space for new, healthy cells.
- Enjoy wholesome natural foods to nourish and fortify the whole.
- Drink plenty of purified water and fresh fruit juices to flush through toxic substances.
- Provide unconditional love and understanding.
- Visit frequently and take on enjoyable outings.

Footnote: *Unconditionally love and forgive those who inflict 'pain' and 'misery' for they inadvertently provide the greatest challenge to discover previously unexploited inner strength and a deeper understanding of the true self.*

CHILLS

Definition

Feverish, cold sensation with a lowered body temperature and shivering.

Emotional aspect

Temporary need to withdraw mentally from life's realities and have time and space for the self.

Reflexes

- Central nervous system, concentrating on the brain reflexes, for stimulation of the hypothalamus, at base of brain, and to naturalise body temperature and centre the mind.
- Endocrine system reflexes, particularly the pituitary, pineal, thymus and adrenal gland reflexes, for emotional control and inner understanding.

Other suggestions

- Seek professional guidance if severe.
- Massage both feet, particularly the toes, with aromatherapy essential oils for inner calm: geranium, ginger.
- Keep the body comfortable.
- Enjoy a warm drink of lemon and honey in hot water.

- Relaxation techniques.
- Bach flower remedies for patience and understanding.

Footnote: *Make time and space for the self, especially during particularly demanding and hectic periods.*

COLIC

Definition

Severe pain due to the spasmodic contraction of the involuntary muscle in bodily tubes, such as the colon, bile duct or uterus.

Emotional aspect

Irritable restlessness, intolerance and vexation with immediate situations.

Reflexes

- See Abdominal Cramp and Colic.

- Concentrate on the liver reflexes to eliminate irritability and intolerance.
- Bile duct, colon or uterine reflexes for the natural expansion and contraction of the ducts.

Other suggestions

- Massage both feet, especially the toes and insteps, with aromatherapy essential oils to pacify the whole: dill diluted in almond oil. Also massage the stomach and back, with clockwise movements.
- Sniff peppermint.
- Apple herb tea with slice of raw apple, peppermint tea, fennel tea.
- Relaxation techniques for inner tranquillity.
- Bach flower remedies to relax and let go.

Footnote: *Something 'good' generally comes from something 'bad'.*

CYST

Definition

A natural, hollow organ (such as the bladder) containing a natural liquid, or an abnormal sac containing unnatural fluid.

Emotional aspect

In its natural state it provides a temporary reservoir for emotions. Imbalances occur when unexpressed painful emotions accumulate and consistently plague thoughts, either consciously or subconsciously.

Reflexes

- The central nervous system for free exchange of progressive thoughts.
- Endocrine system reflexes, especially the pituitary, pineal, thymus and adrenal gland reflexes to release hampering emotions and for emotional balance.
- Liver reflexes to eliminate accumulated emotions.
- Specific reflexes of the affected areas (see the foot chart) to release from the grips of anxiety and to allow the free exchange of emotions.
- Circulatory, lymphatic and urinary system reflexes to encourage free circulation of life-forces and expulsion of all toxic substances.

Other suggestions

- Seek professional guidance.
- Massage both feet and affected reflexes with aromatherapy essential oils to accelerate healing: camomile, clary sage, fennel, geranium, rose, rosemary.

DEATH

Definition

The soul vacates the physical body to return to the spiritual world of truth and love.

Emotional aspect

There is no need to manifest a physical body for the present.

Reflexes

- Prior to death, tremendous comfort and inner peace can be obtained through massaging the feet, easing the transition from the physical to the spiritual realms.
- When the soul leaves the body the feet take on a transparent, smooth, lifeless, plastic appearance as the stresses and strains dissipate, and the impressions of life no longer leave their mark.

Other suggestions

- Before death, reassure the person of your unconditional love for them and deal with any unresolved emotions.
- Feel at ease with the departed.
- Allow them to go in peace by lovingly cutting the chakras and setting them free.

DIZZINESS

See also Loss of Balance

Definition

Either a feeling that objects are spinning around or a subjective rotation. Haziness or unsteadiness, accompanied by anxiety.

Emotional aspect

Fear of acknowledging certain perceptions. Scattered, ungrounded thoughts.

Reflexes

- Central nervous system reflexes, especially the solar plexus reflexes, to centre the mind and calm the nerves.

- Concentrate on the throat, neck, cheek and shoulder reflexes to release from the grips of tension and allow the free flow of essential life-forces.
- Endocrine system reflexes, particularly the pituitary, pineal, thyroid and adrenal gland reflexes for self-confidence, emotional stability and inner strength.
- Circulatory, lymphatic and urinary system reflexes to eliminate toxic substances and to balance the whole.

Other suggestions

- Massage both feet with aromatherapy essential oils to clear the head further: eucalyptus, frankincense, geranium, lavender, peppermint.
- Homoeopathic remedies: Arnica – for early stages; China – when accompanied by nausea and tinnitus. Ruta – to relieve associated eye weakness and strain.
- Relaxation techniques for inner peace.
- Bach flower remedies, especially Rescue Remedy, to still the mind.

FAT

OBESITY

See Digestive System

FATIGUE

Definition

State of weariness that ranges from mental disinclination for effort, tiredness and an absence of energy to a state of total collapse from profound exhaustion due to extreme physical and mental input or distress.

Emotional aspect

'Switching off' due to a lack of interest arising from a loss of control, resistance, or boredom with current circumstances.

Reflexes

- Central nervous system reflexes to alert the senses and revitalise interest.
- Endocrine system reflexes, particularly the pituitary, pineal, thymus and adrenal gland reflexes, to boost enthusiasm by feeling emotionally in control and raising energy levels.
- Neck and shoulder reflexes to release from the grips of anxiety.
- Liver reflexes for the subconscious release of draining emotions so that the whole is injected with enthusiasm.
- Circulatory, lymphatic and urinary system reflexes to rejuvenate the whole with a free exchange of essential life-forces.
- All bodily reflexes, concentrating on the affected areas (see the foot chart), for overall revitalisation.

Other suggestions

- Seek professional guidance if severe.
- Massage both feet and the body with aromatherapy essential oils to further revitalise the whole: bergamot, camomile, clary sage, frankincense, marjoram, vetiver.
- Mental rest through relaxation techniques to rejuvenate mind, body and soul.
- Eat wholesome, natural foods to energise and fuel the whole.
- Vitamin and mineral supplements for increased vitality.
- Bach flower remedies for the ability to cope.
- Relaxation techniques for inner strength.
- Drink plenty of purified fluids and fresh fruit juices.

FEVER

Definition

Unnaturally high temperature, with rapid pulse and respiration rates, dry skin, vomiting and headaches. Excessive changes and destruction of bodily tissue may also occur.

Emotional aspect

Incensed, fuming, letting off steam.

Reflexes

- Central nervous system reflexes, particularly the solar plexus reflexes, to ease tension and put thoughts into perspective.
- Endocrine system reflexes, especially the pituitary, pineal, thymus and adrenal gland reflexes, to lower bodily temperature and reduce inflammatory condition.
- Neck and shoulder reflexes for free energy distribution throughout.
- Respiratory system reflexes to calm respiratory rate.
- Circulatory system reflexes to naturalise the pulse rate.
- Digestive tract reflexes, especially the liver reflexes for inner stability.
- Lymphatic reflexes to eliminate toxic substances.
- All bodily systems on both feet to relax the whole and re-establish equilibrium.

Other suggestions

- Seek professional guidance.
- Massage both feet with aromatherapy essential oils to balance the whole: camomile, eucalyptus, lavender, tea-tree.
- Tepid sponging or lukewarm baths to reduce the fever.
- Drink plenty of purified fluids.
- Apply a natural oil to the skin.
- Relaxation techniques to still the mind.
- Bach flower remedies for inner tranquillity.

FLUID RETENTION

See Oedema

GLANDS

Definition

Special organs which form and secrete fluid, either for use by the body or for excretion.

Emotional aspect

Glands store emotion and encourage self-motivation.

Reflexes

- See Foot Chart for specific references.

Other suggestions

- Massage both feet with aromatherapy essential oils to tone and energise: basil, celery, fennel, grapefruit, lavender, lemongrass, juniper.
- Relaxation techniques for inner harmony.
- Bach flower remedies for a balanced view of life.

Footnote: *Eliminate stagnated emotions that prohibit development and allow energies to flow freely for ongoing progress.*

GLANDULAR DISORDERS

Definition

Inadequate manufacture, secretion, distribution or uptake of secretions due to tension, creating temporary imbalance of certain bodily functions.

Emotional aspect

Lack of motivation or insufficient belief in personal capabilities.

Reflexes

- Central nervous system reflexes, particularly the brain reflexes to stimulate the hypothalamus for a balanced control of all glands.
- Concentrate on all endocrine glands for the natural production and release of secretions.
- For specific reflexes refer to the foot chart for the efficient production and excretion of secretion.
- Circulatory, lymphatic and urinary system reflexes to ease the distribution of hormones and the elimination of by-products of metabolism.

- All bodily reflexes to relax target cells for the efficient uptake and utilisation of all glandular secretions.

Other suggestions

- Seek professional guidance.
- Massage both feet with aromatherapy essential oils to help tone and energise: basil, celery, fennel, grapefruit, lavender, lemongrass, juniper.
- See Glandular Fever.

Footnote: *Thoughts of unconditional love and joy recharge the mind, body and soul with renewed interest and enthusiasm for life.*

GOUT

Definition

A febrile, metabolic disease associated with excessive uric acid in the blood. There are periodic paroxysms of painful inflammation and swellings of joints, especially smaller joints of thumb and big toe, due to urate deposits.

Emotional aspect

Intense desire to be in absolute control. Complete frustration and intolerance. Feeling insecure particularly with own perceptions, reasoning and intellect.

Reflexes

- Central nervous system reflexes, concentrating on all reflexes, to ease extreme pain and for intuitive, intellectual control and understanding. Gently massage the afflicted big toe or auric space around it if it is too painful to touch.
- Endocrine system, especially the pituitary, thymus and adrenal gland reflexes, to reduce inflammation and for emotional security.
- Joint reflexes, particularly the neck, shoulder, thumb and big toe reflexes, for increased flexibility and to reduce the swelling of the affected joints.

- Liver reflexes to release stored emotions and for natural energy to revitalise the whole.
- Circulatory, lymphatic and urinary reflexes to eliminate all toxic deposits and encourage free flow of life-forces.

Other suggestions

- Seek professional guidance.
- Massage both feet, especially the toes and heels, with aromatherapy essential oils to assist in reducing pain and discomfort: basil, birch, pine, thyme.
- Eat wholesome, natural foods avoiding red meat, alcohol, refined products, chocolates, preservatives and colourants.
- Apply heat to the swollen joints to ease discomfort and rigidity.
- Homoeopathic remedies: Aconite – to reduce acute pain; Belladonna – to ease hot, swollen, tender joints; Colchicum – for swollen big toe; Urtica urens – to relieve intense burning and irritability.
- Relaxation techniques to ease the mind.
- Bach flower remedies for self-control and inner understanding.

Footnote: *Control comes from within through feeling good about the self and life in general.*

GROWTHS

Definition

Unnatural development of the tissue and cells.

Emotional aspect

Built-up emotional hurts, disappointments or resentments.

Reflexes

- Central nervous system reflexes to make space for thoughts of understanding and forgiveness.
- Endocrine system to balance emotions.

- Affected area reflex(es) to relax from the grips of tension, so that malformed cells can be taken away and replaced by new healthy cells.
- Liver reflexes for the release of built-up emotions.
- Circulatory, lymphatic and urinary system reflexes for the elimination of toxic substances.
- All bodily reflexes on both feet for overall health.

Other suggestions
- See Stress
- Seek professional advice if necessary.

Footnote: *'Good' and 'bad' experiences of life, if accepted with love and understanding, are a blessing rather than a curse.*

HALITOSIS

See Bad Breath

HAY FEVER

See Allergies

HERNIA

Definition

Rupture and protrusion of part of an internal organ through a weakened structure.

Cerebral hernia: protrusion of the brain through an opening in the skull.

Femoral hernia: a loop of the intestine protrudes through the femoral canal.

Hiatus hernia: part of the stomach protrudes through the oesophageal opening in the diaphragm. Also known as a diaphragmatic hernia.

Incisional hernia: at the site of an old wound. Also called a ventral hernia.

Inguinal hernia: the protrusion of the intestine through the inguinal canal.

Irreducible hernia: a protrusion that cannot be replaced by manipulation.

Reducible hernia: a protrusion that can be reduced through manipulation.

Strangulated hernia: the circulation becomes constricted causing complications.

Umbilical hernia: the bowel protrudes through the umbilical ring.

Vaginal hernia: the bladder or rectum protrude into the vagina.

Emotional aspect

A breach of harmonious relationships, excessive strain, feeling overstretched, or being prevented from expressing true creativity.

Reflexes

- Central nervous system reflexes, especially the big and fourth toes, to enhance general communication and to strengthen relationships.
- Endocrine system reflexes for emotional harmony.
- Shoulder reflexes to relax the musculature.
- Liver reflexes to release extreme emotions.
- The reflex of the hernia to relax pressure and allow the protruding tissue to return to its natural position.

Other suggestions

- Seek professional advice.
- Massage both feet with aromatherapy essential oils for inner peace: basil, geranium, cypress, hyssop, lavender, rosemary. Hiatus hernia – coriander, fennel, ginger, rosemary; Incisional hernia – ginger, lavender, lemon, neroli, rose; Inguinal hernia – basil, ginger, lavender, rosemary.
- Relaxation techniques for total harmony.
- Bach flower remedies for inner calm and understanding.

HIRSUTISM

ALOPECIA

Definition

Hair is made up of fine filaments growing from follicles within the skin.

Alopecia: total or partial hair loss due to extreme tension or shock. Believed to be hereditary
Hirsutism: excessive bodily hair.
Tension: impinges on the hair follicles, weakens hair and causes it to break off. Long term, new growth is prevented due to lack of space within the follicle.

Emotional aspect

Hair provides strength and emotional protection thereby reducing vulnerability to outside forces.

Alopecia: profound distress and anxiety from not coping with the demands of life. The pressure of trying too hard to be in control.
Hirsutism: covering up or protecting the true emotions.
Tension: scalp eruptions due to emotional suppression or disturbances.

Reflexes

Reflexology naturalises hair growth, calms overactivity and speeds up underactivity.

- Central nervous system reflexes, especially the big and second toes, for improved self-esteem and to trust own intuition.
- Endocrine reflexes, concentrating on all reflexes, for hormonal balance.
- Hair follicle reflexes, throughout both feet, either to strengthen hair growth for added protection or to reduce excessive hair growth to break down defences.

Other suggestions

- New Era Laboratory Limited (for hair analysis), Marfleet, Hull HU9 SNJ.

- Seek the advice of a trichologist.
- Massage both feet and the scalp with aromatherapy essential oils for healthy hair growth: carrot, eucalyptus, lavender, lemon, parsley, rosemary.
- Wash the hair daily and massage the scalp thoroughly with professionally recommended shampoo, to release physical tension.
- Enjoy wholesome, natural foods, preferably raw, for strong healthy hair fibres.
- Relaxation techniques to ease the mind.
- Vitamin A and C supplements.
- Reduce alcohol intake if hair tangles easily.
- For excessive hair loss during pregnancy, stressful periods and antibiotic treatment, chop up 50 g nettle and 100 g burdock root, mix in 500 ml rum, store for 8–10 days, then rub on scalp and drink!
- For nits, add tea-tree oil to the shampoo.
- For brittle hair massage two tablespoonfuls of warm jojoba oil into the scalp and leave on for half an hour.
- For oily hair use Bryonia (1/6th potency) homoeopathic remedy.
- For premature greying hair take the Chinese herb, he shou wu.
- For itchy scalp wash with tea-tree oil blended with cedarwood shampoo.
- For split ends, cut off, avoid hair driers, apply warmed olive oil to the hair ends, then wrap in a towel.

INCURABLE DISEASE

Definition

No known chemical, physical or material cure for a particular disease.

Emotional aspect

Hopelessness from misguided beliefs that no cure is available for certain diseases. However, treatment in the form of drugs, natural therapy, surgery, nutrition and exercise can sufficiently relieve the physical symptoms for there to be a shift in attitude and inner healing to take place.

Reflexes

- Central nervous system reflexes, concentrating on all reflexes, to elevate the level of consciousness and release social conditioning.
- Endocrine system reflexes, spending time on all reflexes, for inner strength and emotional understanding.
- Specific reflexes of the affected area to release from the grips of fear and anxiety to make space for healing.
- Circulatory, lymphatic and urinary system reflexes to flush through and eliminate toxic substances as well as old beliefs.
- All bodily reflexes on both feet for overall harmony.

Other suggestions

- The power of the mind is so great that **any** limiting belief systems can be **immediately** overcome by a shift in the thought process, **provided** there is a genuine desire to improve.

INFLAMMATION

Definition

A series of physical changes in bodily tissue, with heat, swelling, pain and redness.

Emotional aspect

Incensed, outrageous anger. Highly inflammable emotions that ignite when security is threatened.

Reflexes

- As for Fever.
- Give particular attention to the affected areas (see foot chart) for inner harmony.

Other suggestions
- See Fevers.

INFLUENZA

Definition

Acute infectious febrile disorder due to one of a variety of viral strains, often in epidemic proportion.

Emotional aspect

Submission to social depression, insecurity and negativity from conditioned social belief systems. Longing for unconditional love, approval and reassurance.

Reflexes
- As for Fever and Chills.
- Concentrate on the central nervous system reflexes, especially the big and second toes, to centre the mind and release inhibiting belief systems and overwhelming feelings.

Other suggestions
- See Fever and Chills.
- Homoeopathic remedies: Aconite – for the early stages to reduce rigors, fevers, chills: Arsenicum – to relieve exhaustion, weakness and prostration; Bryonia – to ease a dry cough, fever and muscular aches.

Footnote: *Intuition lovingly shows the way to understanding the meaning of life.*

INJURIES

Definition

Hurt or harm due to external forces cutting, tearing or bruising bodily tissue.

Emotional aspect

Wounded feelings and damaged pride. Subconsciously hurting
and punishing the self due to frustration, guilt or resistance to the
natural flow of life. The position on the body and feet is
significant.

Head and toes: battered thoughts.
Throat and necks of toes: hurtful expressions.
Chest and upper arms and balls of feet: bruised emotions.
Upper abdomen and lower arms and upper insteps: blocked
activity.
Lower abdomen and hands and lower insteps: hurtful
communication.
Pelvis, legs and feet and heels: obstructed movements.

Reflexes

- As for Pain.
- Concentrate on the muscular reflexes, especially the neck
  and shoulder reflexes, to reduce spasm and discomfort.

Other suggestions

- If severe, seek professional guidance.
- Initially apply a cold compress to contract the blood vessels,
  reduce swelling, prevent inflammation, ease the pain and
  decrease the collection of blood.
- Twelve hours later, apply heat to dilate the capillaries to
  increase the blood flow, reduce the spasm and nourish the
  tissues.
- For open wounds apply seaweed fluid or cayenne powder to
  immediately stop bleeding.
- Iron a cabbage leaf and apply to the afflicted area.
- Massage both feet with aromatherapy essential oils to
  accelerate healing: camomile, grapefruit, lavender, rosemary,
  tea-tree.
- Bach flower remedies, especially Rescue Remedy, for inner
  calm.

Footnote: *Wisdom is acquired by going through life's experiences
and learning that there are many ways of doing things. Be kind to
the self!*

MALARIA

Definition

Febrile disease caused by the injected parasite of the female genus Anopheles mosquito. Periodic attacks start with a shivering fit, followed by high fever and profuse sweating.

Emotional aspect

Anger for feeling ill at ease. Deep insecurity resulting in obsessiveness. Wanting total control.

Reflexes

- As for Fever.
- Concentrate on the splenic reflexes to reduce fever and elminate obsessive behaviour.

Other suggestions

- Seek professional guidance.
- Massage both feet, concentrating on the toes and insteps, with aromatherapy essential oils to calm the whole: eucalyptus, lavender, thyme.
- Apply neat lavender oil to the bites.
- Tepid sponging or lukewarm baths to reduce fever.
- Bed-rest.
- Drink plenty of purified fluids until able to manage small portions of wholesome, nourishing food.
- Vitamin and mineral supplements for increased vitality.

Footnote: *Resistance creates havoc, whereas faith in the cosmic order of life provides knowledge and resources for inner strength and control.*

NAIL BITING AND TEARING

Definition

Chewing or stripping the horny covering on the tips of the fingers, thumbs and toes.

Emotional aspect

Vulnerability due to total frustration and uncertainty ripping the very essence of one's being. Eating away at the self. The digit/s affected is/are significant.

Thumb and big toe: indecisive thoughts tearing away at the intellect and intuition. Extreme concern.

Index finger and second toe: feelings frustrated by thoughts that are ripping the self apart. Shifting the blame on to others.

Third finger and third toe: angry, destructive thoughts and actions.

Ring finger and fourth toe: unpleasant thoughts searing away at relationships and communication.

Little finger and toe: insecure thoughts eroding mobility and expansion.

Reflexes

- As for Nervous Disorders.
- Concentrate on the hand or feet reflexes for free expression and mobility.

Other suggestions

- Massage both feet, especially the toes and ankle-bones, with aromatherapy essential oils to stimulate the growth of strong, healthy nails: grapefruit, lavender, lemon, rosemary.
- Regular pedicures and manicures. To look good is to feel good!
- Use fingers for the creative expression of the true self.
- Stretch the toes wide apart for open-mindedness.
- Put bitter aloes on nails to prevent biting!
- Relaxation techniques for inner calm.

NARCOLEPSY

Definition

Uncontrollable desire to sleep.

Emotional aspect

Fear of not being able to cope with the reality of life.

Reflexes

- As for Nervous Disorders.
- Concentrate on all reflexes on both feet for overall confidence and energy.

Other suggestions

- See Nervous Disorders.

Footnote: *Find and become involved in an all-consuming interest in life!*

NUMBNESS

Definition

Temporary lack of feeling or motion.

Emotional aspect

Momentarily withholding love, joy and consideration by mentally switching off!

Reflexes

- As for Nervous Disorders
- Concentrate on all central nervous system reflexes to regain mental control.

Other suggestions

- Massage both feet and the affected area with aromatherapy essential oils to assist with the return of sensation: basil, camomile, eucalyptus, lemon, neroli, rosemary.
- Bach flower remedies to overcome temporary blockage.
- Relaxation techniques for inner peace.

Footnote: *Giving is receiving, so unconditionally share love and joy.*

OEDEMA

FLUID RETENTION

SWELLING

Definition

Swollen tissue due to the effusion of excessive fluids into the affected area. Pitting occurs when pressure is applied locally.

Cardiac oedema: due to heart failure.
Famine oedema: deficiency in the diet.
Lymphatic oedema: blockage in lymphatic system.
Pulmonary oedema: effusion of fluid into lungs.
Venous oedema: obstruction in veins.
Renal oedema: due to nephritis.

Emotional aspect

Feeling trapped and yet afraid to let go for fear of losing something. Weighed down by life's responsibilities, with little or no space for pleasurable pursuits.

Reflexes

- Concentrate on all central nervous system reflexes to give free reign to the thought process.
- Endocrine systems reflexes, spending time on all reflexes, to release trapped emotions.
- Reflexes of the affected areas to relax tissue, encourage absorption of excess fluids and re-establish a healthy cycle of life-forces.
- Liver reflexes to release accumulated resentment.
- Circulatory, lymphatic and urinary reflexes to eliminate excess fluid.
- All bodily reflexes to revitalise the whole.

Other suggestions

- Seek professional guidance.
- Massage both feet, especially the affected reflexes, with aromatherapy essential oils to help drain away excess fluids: cypress, ginger, lavender.

- Ice compresses to ease the swelling.
- Spring-clean everything! Start with the house. Throw or give away anything that has not been used or worn for six months or more. By letting go physically, it is easier to let go emotionally!
- Flush the body out with fresh fruit juice and raw vegetables for a few days. Excessive urination and diarrhoea are an excellent sign of releasing toxic wastes and emotions!
- Relaxation techniques for total release.
- Rest with feet elevated, if the oedema is in legs.
- Keep as active as possible and enjoy everything you do!
- Bach flower remedies to let go with love and understanding.

PAIN

Definition

Sensation of physical or emotional distress and suffering that travels along fine nerve endings through the peripheral nerves to the brain indicating discomfort or disease. Referred pain is felt at a distance from the distressed area.

Emotional aspect

Resisting the flow of life due to fear, anxiety or self-inflicted guilt. The position on the body indicates the perception:

Head pain: out of control.
Neck and shoulder pain: hurt expressions, lack of flexibility.
Arm pains: restricted and restrained.
Chest pains: painful emotions, hurt within the environment.
Abdominal pain: activities and communications cause personal grief.
Leg pains: fear of a painful future or feeling very insecure. Resistance in moving ahead.

Reflexes

- Central nervous system reflexes, especially the solar plexus reflexes, for courage and understanding.

- Endocrine system reflexes, particularly the pituitary, pineal, thymus and adrenal gland reflexes, for emotional strength.
- Liver reflexes to release old hurts.
- Circulatory, lymphatic and urinary system reflexes to eliminate toxic substances and for the free distribution of vibrant energy.
- Specific reflex (see the foot chart) and all bodily reflexes to ease the whole.

Other suggestions

- Massage both feet and the painful area itself with aromatherapy essential oils for their analgesic properties: clove, eucalyptus, thyme mixed with lanolin and rosewater.
- Cool application to numb the sensation or heat to dilate the blood vessels and nourish the affected area.
- Breathe into the discomfort and concentrate on taking large deep breaths.
- Relaxation techniques for peace of mind.
- Bach flower Rescue Remedy to calm emotions.

Footnote: *Relax and go with the natural flow and excitement of life!*

PARASITES

See also Worms (Digestive system)

Definition

An animal or vegetable organism that lives and thrives upon or within another for its nourishment.

Emotional aspect

Allowing others to dominate and draw upon resources.

Reflexes

- As for Nervous Disorders.
- Concentrate on the circulatory, lymphatic and urinary system reflexes for the natural elimination of unwanted substances.

Other suggestions:

- See Worms and Digestive Disorders.

PYORRHOEA

Definition

Discharge of pus.

Emotional aspect

Angry indecisiveness outpouring from the very core of the being.

Reflexes

- As for Fever.
- Concentrate on the specific reflexes for the afflicted areas (see the foot chart) to encourage the elimination of toxic substances so that healthy vibrant cells can develop.

Other suggestions

- See Fever.

Footnote: *Life is an ongoing cycle of love and joy.*

SNORING

Definition

Hoarse rattling or grunting noise interrupting breath, especially during sleep, but also during the alpha state of relaxation.

Emotional aspect

Release of deeply suppressed emotions that have had no other outlet.

Reflexes

- As for Nervous Disorders.
- Concentrate on the liver reflexes for the natural outlet of deeply suppressed emotions and irritating substances.

Other suggestions

- Massage both feet with aromatherapy essential oils to help relax musculature: bergamot, cypress, frankincense, lemon, lavender, rosemary.
- Relaxation techniques to create a natural outlet of suppressed emotions.
- Wholesome, natural foods to ease digestion.
- Avoid excessive alcohol.

Footnote: *Express true emotions openly and lovingly.*

SORES

Definition

Extreme tenderness of the skin, sometimes with a break in the superficial and subcutaneous tissue, which may become infected.

Emotional aspect

Suppressed hurts coming to the surface after having been concealed.

Reflexes

- As for Skin Disorders.
- Concentrate on the specific reflexes of the affected areas to promote healing.

Other suggestions

- See Pain and Skin Disorders.

SPLEEN

Definition

An extremely vascular lymphoid organ, situated below the stomach, that manufactures lymphocytes and breaks down the red blood cells at the end of their cycle.

Emotional aspect

A relaxed and balanced approach to life and all activities because feeling intuitively in control and making appropriate responses.

Reflexes

Splenic reflex on the left foot only. Soft, palpable mound occupying the upper right quadrant of the left instep. Massage to naturalise functioning and to encourage a more relaxed approach to life.

Other suggestions

• Maintain a balanced lifestyle.

Footnote: *Everything pursued with unconditional love and joy is always 'perfect'.*

SPLENIC DISORDERS

Definition

Interference with the natural functioning of the spleen prevents the efficient manufacture of lymphocytes and the breakdown of red blood cells.

Emotional aspect

Preoccupied and haunted by a precise approach to activities. Obsessive type of personality.

Reflexes

The splenic reflex swells particularly during a malarial attack.

• Central nervous system reflexes to calm the mind.
• Endocrine system reflexes for emotional understanding.
• Splenic reflexes to nurture and balance.
• Liver reflexes to release stored anxiety.

- Digestive reflexes, concentrating on the colon reflexes, for flexibility and adaptability.
- Lymphatic system reflexes to release the toxic build-up.

Other suggestions

- Seek professional guidance.
- Massage both feet, concentrating on the toes and left instep, with aromatherapy essential oils to further pacify the whole: camomile, clary sage, lavender, lemon, marjoram, neroli, nutmeg, pettigraine, vetiver.
- Relaxation techniques for peace of mind.
- Enjoy wholesome, natural food to fortify the whole.
- A balanced lifestyle.
- Bach flower remedies for inner calm.

Footnote: *A balanced approach to life allows everything to fall into perspective.*

STIFFNESS

Definition

Rigidity. Incapable of flexibility, usually of the muscles.

Emotional aspect

Uncompromising, obstinate, unyielding and unbending in attitude. Need to feel in control at all times.

Reflexes

- As for Muscular Disorders.
- Concentrate on all bodily reflexes for overall ease.

Other suggestions

- See Muscular Disorders.

Footnote: *Ultimate control comes from feeling secure and being able to adapt to everything and anything.*

STUTTERING

Definition

Repetition of words, especially the initial consonants.

Emotional aspect

Vulnerability and self-consciousness at not being able to express the true self.

Reflexes

- Central nervous system reflexes, especially the brain and solar plexus reflexes, to make space for self-confidence.
- Endocrine system reflexes, especially the pituitary, pineal, thymus and adrenal reflexes, for emotional strength and understanding.
- Neck, throat and shoulder reflexes to release from the grips of anxiety for free expression.
- Liver reflexes to eliminate pent-up anxiety.
- Circulatory, lymphatic and urinary system reflexes to eliminate toxic substances for the free flow of energy.

Other suggestions

- Seek professional guidance.
- Massage both feet, concentrating on the toes and necks of the toes, with aromatherapy essential oils to relax the whole musculature: bergamot, camomile, geranium, grapefruit, lavender, rosemary.
- Relaxation techniques for inner calm.
- Alexander technique to realign the whole naturally.
- Bach flower remedies, particularly Rescue Remedy at times of extreme anxiety.

STRESS

DISTRESS

Definition

Stress is an essential component for the balance in life. If the balance is tipped then strain, tension, hassle, anxiety, oppression and pressure are experienced. These are manifested in feeling burdened, wary, tense, traumatised, worried or concerned. Distress is intangible. It cannot be seen, heard, tasted, smelt, felt, measured but it can be detected through physical, mental and emotional bodily changes.

Emotional aspect

A clear mind manifests a clear body. Control is influenced by feelings, thoughts and actions. Distress does not enter the body, but is an outward manifestation of inner feelings, emotions and thoughts.

Reflexes

- Refer to the foot chart for specific areas.

Other suggestions

- Seek professional advice.
- Feel committed to life with an ability and willingness to be involved.
- Enjoy challenges expecting to change and welcome that change for personal development.
- Massage both feet with aromatherapy essential oils to enhance inner tranquillity: camomile, fennel, geranium, lavender, lemon, rosemary.
- Relaxation techniques.
- Bach flower remedies for the ability to cope.

Footnote: *Live life to the full – don't allow a death sentence to bring you to your senses!*

SWELLING

Definition

Tissue that is raised from the surrounding surface.

Emotional aspect

The surfacing of old emotional hurts or inflated belief systems.

Reflexes

- As for Oedema.
- Spend time on the reflexes of affected areas (see the foot chart) to encourage the free exchange of essential life-forces and toxic substances.

Other suggestions

- See Oedema.
- Ice compress to ease the swelling.

THRUSH

See Candida Albicans

TUMOURS

Definition

The growth of malformed tissue that has been deprived of its essential nutrients and inhibited by the build-up of toxic wastes, due to tension.

Emotional aspect

Accumulated fear, anxiety and resentment at not being able to express true feelings, especially those of anger, frustration and deep hurt.

Reflexes

- As for Stress.
- Through the relaxation of the reflexology massage malformed cells are absorbed at the end of their cycle by lymph vessels and are replaced with new, vibrant cells in harmonious surroundings. Billions of new cells are formed within the body every second, which effectively means that the body has a complete overhaul on a regular basis!
- Concentrate on the reflexes of the affected areas to promote the healing process.

Other suggestions

- See Stress.
- Join a local self-help group.
- Relaxation techniques (pages 000) to release the past.
- Eat wholesome, natural food for vibrant, new cells.
- Drink plenty purified fluids to flush through toxic wastes.
- Use motivational tapes and books to accelerate the healing.

Footnote: *Live for the here and now – the past is over whilst the future represents present joys magnified.*

WEAKNESS

Definition

Lack of physical or emotional strength or power. Easily defeated.

Emotional aspect

Depletion of energy from the strain of trying to control everything and everyone.

Reflexes

- As for Fatigue.

Other suggestions

- See Fatigue.

Footnote: *Provide space for the mind, body and soul to feel the natural flow of universal energy and vitality.*

WOUNDS

See Injuries

*A*PPENDIX 1

BACH FLOWER REMEDIES

Aversion to company
Impatiens: For patience and ability to work with others.
Mimulus: To reduce fears of everyday life.
Water violet: Overcome the need to be alone.

Apathy
Clematis: To bring dreamers and escapists back to present.
Wild rose: To provide enthusiasm for life.

Cleanser
Crab apple: For self-acceptance.

Day dreaming
Clematis: To acknowledge reality.
Honeysuckle: To release the past.

Depression
Gentian: For personal encouragement.
Mustard: To raise the spirits and give hope.

Despair
Gorse: For faith and belief in success.
Rock rose: For courage and hope.
Sweet chestnut: To release anguish and make anything possible.

Domination
Chicory: To allow space for self and others.
Heather: For faith in the self.
Vervain: To accept others.

Embittered
Holly: To release life's vexations.
Willow: For enlightened perceptions.

Exhausted

Olive:	To provide inner strength.
Hornbeam:	For the ability to cope.
Vervain:	To acknowledge others.
Clematis:	Enjoyment of the present.

Fault-finding in others

Beech:	Acceptance of others.
Chicory:	To give space to others.
Holly:	To release envy, jealousy and other vexations.
Impatiens:	For patience to work alongside others.
Willow:	To release resentment and accept equality of life.

Fault-finding with the self

Rock water:	For self-acceptance.

Fear

Aspen:	For faith and reasoning.

Fixed ideas and opinions

Beech:	For tolerance to look at other points of view.
Rock water:	To release the self from self-imposed shackles.
Vervain:	To accept others for who and what they are.
Vine:	To make space for everyone.

Greed

Chicory:	To allow others to be themselves.
Vervain:	To release others from possessive grips.
Vine:	For security with the self.

Hate

Holly:	To release intense emotions.
Willow:	For acceptance of the self and others.

Hopelessness

Gorse:	For hope and belief in success.
Rock rose:	For deep faith and unconditional love.
Sweet chestnut:	To release anguish and make everything bearable.

Idealistic
Beech: For tolerance of life.
Impatiens: For patience and acceptance of others.
Rock water: For self-acceptance.
Vervain: To release the need to change everything.

Impatience
Impatiens: For patience and acceptance of others.
Chestnut bud: To see life's opportunities.

Insanity
Cherry plum: For strength of mind.
Clematis: To be brought down to earth!

Intolerance
Impatiens: For patience and ability to work with others.
Beech: For tolerance.
Vervain: To accept others.
Water violet: For enjoyment of company.

Jealousy
Holly: To release jealousy.

Lack of concentration
Clematis: To bring back to the present.
White chestnut: For peace of mind and the release of unwanted thoughts.

Lack of confidence
Cerato: For decisiveness.
Larch: For self-confidence.
Scleranthus: To instil certainty.

Lack of vitality
Agrimony: For honest openmindedness.
Centaury: For self-assurance and assertiveness.
Clematis: For energy for the here and now.
Mimulus: For confidence and faith.

Loneliness
Heather: For self-acceptance.
Agrimony: For inner peace and understanding.

Chicory:	To create space for the self.
Mimulus:	For faith and joy.

Misguided

Centaury:	For self-assurance.
Cerato:	For self-confidence.
Walnut:	For self-protection.

Nervous breakdown

Cherry plum:	For strength of mind.
Oak:	For inner strength.
Vervain:	For belief in others.
Scleranthus:	For decisiveness.

Obsession

Cherry plum:	For clarity of mind.
Oak:	For inner strength.
Vervain:	To believe in others.
Clematis:	To accept the reality of life.

Possessiveness

Chicory:	To release others.
Heather:	For self-acceptance.

Procrastination

Larch:	For self-confidence.
Mimulus:	For faith and hope.
Scleranthus:	For decisiveness.

Restlessness

Agrimony:	To accept the true self.
Scleranthus:	For decisive action.
Impatiens:	For patience.
Vervain:	For acceptance of others.

Self-centred

Chicory:	To provide space for the self and others.
Heather:	For inner peace and understanding.
Willow:	To release resentment.

Self-hate

Crab apple:	For acceptance of the self.

| *Cerato:* | For self-confidence. |
| *Rock water:* | For self-assurance. |

Self-pity

Chicory:	To create space for others.
Heather:	For inner peace and understanding.
Willow:	To release resentments.

Shock

Rescue Remedy:	For emergencies, stress, shock and anxiety.
Star of Bethlehem:	To provide comfort and reassurance.
Rock rose:	For faith and understanding.

Suicidal

Agrimony:	To accept the true self.
Aspen:	To release unknown fears.
Cherry plum:	For strength of mind.
Clematis:	For acceptance of reality.
Mimulus:	For faith and understanding.

Tension

Beech:	For tolerance of others.
Impatiens:	For patience and ability to work with others.
Rock water:	For self-acceptance.
Vervain:	For ability to relax and let go.
Vine:	For faith in universal order.

Weariness

Centaury:	For self-control and confidence.
Hornbeam:	For the ability to cope.
Olive:	For inner strength.
Wild rose:	For determination.

Worry

Red chestnut:	To release over-concern for others.
Heather:	To release fear of being alone.
Agrimony:	For confidence to express true self.
White chestnut:	To ease the mind.

𝒶PPENDIX 2

REFLEXOLOGY AND VIBRATIONAL THERAPY

All toe pads, specifically the big toe

Colour:	Purple, indigo, violet, white.
Properties:	Highest vibration and greatest wisdom.
	Heightens intuitive thoughts and spirituality.
	Transmutes desires from thoughts into reality.
	For understanding life and the self.
Healing:	Soothes the nerves and clears the mind.
Gems:	Amethyst, white diamond, lapis lazuli.
Musical note:	Indigo: A and violet: B
Music:	Gregorian chants.
	Neptune and venus music by Holst.
Food:	Beetroot, purple grapes.
Flower:	Violet.

Necks of toes

Colour:	Turquoise/blue.
Properties:	Two-way expression.
	Connects the physical and etherical bodies.
Healing:	Cooling, soothing astringent.
Gems:	Turquoise, blue sapphires, blue lace.
Musical note:	G
Music:	Ave Maria by Schubert.
	Crystal Cave by Upper Astral.
Food:	Blueberries.
Flower:	Bluebell.

Balls of feet and second toes

Colour:	Green.
Properties:	Feelings of renewal of life.
Healing:	Rejuvenates the whole and makes space for expansion.
Gems:	Emerald, jade, malachite.
Musical note:	F
Music:	Claire de Lune by Debussy.
	Pan Flute music.

Food:	Leafy vegetables and green fruits.
Nature:	Leaves and grass.

Upper half of the instep and third toes

Colour:	Yellow.
Properties:	Stimulates the logical mind and reasoning powers.
	Self-control through inspiring the higher faculties.
Healing:	Purifies and radiates the whole.
Gems:	Citrine, topaz, yellow diamonds.
Musical note:	E
Music:	Piano Concerto No. 26 by Mozart.
	Kitaro Ki by Kitaro.
Food:	Yellow peppers, mustard, turmeric.
Flower:	Daffodil.

Lower half of the instep and fourth toes

Colour:	Orange.
Properties:	Assimilation, distribution, circulation and elimination.
Healing:	Physically and mentally energising.
	Powerful tonic effect.
Gems:	Orange citrines, amber.
Musical note:	D
Music:	Hungarian Dance No. 5 by Brahms.
	Waterfall Music by Paul Warner.
Food:	Oranges, carrots, mangos.
Flower:	Marigold.

Heels and fifth toes

Colour:	Red
Properties:	The densest energy.
	Provides energy and vitality.
	Base from which to develop.
Healing:	Uplifting and inspires confidence.
Gems:	Ruby, red garnets.
Musical note:	C
Music:	March Militaire by Schubert.
	Mars Music by Holst.
Food:	Raspberries.
Flower:	Poppy.